MANAGING CHILDREN WITH PSYCHIATRIC PROBLEMS

MANAGING CHILDREN WITH PSYCHIATRIC PROBLEMS

Edited by
PROFESSOR M ELENA GARRALDA

Academic Unit of Child and Adolescent Psychiatry
St Mary's Hospital Medical School
London W2 1PG

Published by the BMJ Publishing Group
Tavistock Square, London WC1H 9JR

British Library Cataloguing in Publication Data
A catalogue record for this book is available from the British Library
ISBN 0–7279–0788–3

Typeset, printed in Great Britain by
Latimer Trend & Company Ltd, Plymouth

Contents

v

Preface

For many doctors child psychiatric practice is still a little known area of medicine. Clinicians are often well aware of the relevance of psychological issues for children's health, but they may feel at a loss about how to take effective action and how to explain to families and children the work of child psychiatrists at the point of specialist referral. This book aims to help paediatricians and other doctors to address the psychiatric aspects of children's health problems.

There is now ample evidence attesting to the public health importance of child psychiatric disturbance. Not only are behaviour problems and psychiatric disorders present in a substantial proportion of children in the general population but they can cause considerable handicap to the children by disrupting their development and can lead to considerable suffering for the children and their families. Moreover, many of these disorders show considerable continuity throughout childhood and adolescence.

In recent years it has become clear that children's mental health problems are highly relevant to the work of general practitioners and paediatricians. Many children are brought to their general practitioner and paediatrician with primary psychological symptoms, but even more have psychiatric disturbance as a background factor that contributes to somatic presentations, and psychiatric disorder is probably an important reason for frequent attendance of children to general practice. This is likely to be caused, in part at least, by parents' lack of confidence in dealing with somatic symptoms as an extension of the difficulties they have in handling their child's emotions and behaviour. A helpful consultation with the doctor can be perceived as a needed source of support in the parental role.

There are a few books available that describe the main psychiatric disorders of children in a way that is helpful for paediatricians and general practitioners. However, there are hardly any publications that provide a succinct account of the specific treatment techniques used by child psychiatrists and that may be modified for use by other clinicians. This book should help to fill that gap.

viii

The first part of the book describes how to identify psychiatric problems in children and gives an overview of types of treatment. The evidence supporting the efficacy of these treatments is discussed and guidelines are given for referral to child psychiatry. The second part outlines the most commonly used techniques. Therapies range from the more traditional and clinically tested psychotherapies, such as individual psychotherapy, to the more recently developed but already well established behaviour and family therapy techniques. The chapters on medication and inpatient units address treatments used for only a small proportion of disturbed children, but which are essential components of the service provided by child psychiatry. Readers will see that several different treatments may be effective for individual problems and that treatments are not mutually exclusive. Some of the advantages and disadvantages of different treatment methods are discussed. All the authors are based in the United Kingdom and the book therefore draws heavily on British child psychiatric practice. Contributors are highly experienced in the treatments discussed and, as in the other sections of the book, they provide clear descriptions and sometimes also helpful accounts of personal practice.

As indicated in the overview, most disturbed children are not referred to child psychiatrists. This is partly because there are not enough child psychiatry specialists and services, but also because disturbance in childhood may be closely linked to other medical, social, and educational problems, amelioration of which may need to take primary place in treatment. In these cases, child psychiatrists can usefully share their expertise in liaison or consultation work with those addressing primary difficulties. The third part of the book outlines examples of consultation and liaison work carried out by child psychiatrists. General principles as well as specific liaison work, including paediatric and court work in relation to parenting breakdown and delinquency, are described.

The third part also deals with two issues of special relevance in the current climate of change in health services. The chapter on the organisation of child psychiatric services places a particular emphasis on the methodology for evaluating and improving services, taking into account new audit initiatives and the increased need for service accountability. In line with the current impetus on health promotion and disease prevention, the section on preventive aspects gives an outline of initiatives carried out in the mental health discipline and of the role of child psychiatrists and other mental health professionals in this emergent but important topic.

The book has not addressed specifically the treatment needs of children and youngsters with problems such as autism or learning difficulties. Behaviour problems are common in these children and can be improved by the various treatment techniques outlined in the book, although some methods, especially behaviour modification and consultation work, are particularly appropriate.

The aim of this book is to provide readable, informative, and interesting accounts of child psychiatric treatments that will be of practical use for paediatricians but also to others dealing with children's mental health problems, including general practitioners, psychiatric trainees, teachers, and social workers. It should aid in the referral of the more disturbed children to specialist services, and it should also offer useful treatment strategies for clinicians.

M E Garralda
April 1993

PART I
OVERVIEW

1. Identifying psychiatric disorders in children

John Pearce

Introduction

Children who have a psychiatric disorder are often seen as being difficult rather than disturbed, and the significance of the emotion or the behaviour may easily be missed. The distinction between "normal" and pathological behaviour is important because reassurance is appropriate in the first case and dangerous in the latter.

A psychiatric disorder can be classified as anomalous behaviour, emotions, or thought processes (the three main aspects of mental functioning) that are so prolonged or severe, or both, that they interfere with everyday life and are a handicap for the child or those who care for the child. The child's stage of development and the sociocultural context in which the disorder occurs must also be taken into account (box 1).

Box 1—Definition of childhood psychiatric disorder

- Anomalies in the child's behaviour, emotion, or thoughts
- Persistent—for at least two weeks
- Severe enough to interfere with the child's everyday life
- A handicap to the child, or the carers, or both
- Taking account of the child's stage of development
- Taking account of the sociocultural context.

Rarely, a child's mental state may lead to behaviour so bizarre or extreme that it only has to occur once to be regarded as abnormal. Deliberate self injury or delusions are good examples of this.

Child psychiatric disorder, as defined above, has a one year prevalence of roughly 10% in the general population, which is much the same as it is for adults. This rate is influenced by several risk and protective factors.

3

Risk factors for psychiatric disorders in children

Child risk factors

Surveillance for psychiatric disorder is assisted by knowing the main factors that increase the risk. The most important intrinsic or child based influences that put a child at risk are given in box 2. Most children with a psychiatric disorder will have been unfavourably influenced by more than just a single risk factor. Each of the risk factors interacts with others in such a way that the total adversity is more than the sum of the individual factors. Thus, a 10 year old boy with epilepsy and learning difficulties may have no problems until he is teased for being slow at school, which results in low self esteem, and that in turn interferes with his motivation to learn.

Box 2—Child risk factors for psychiatric disorder

- Low IQ—risk as high as 40% for children with severe learning difficulties
- Difficult temperament
- Physical illness—greatly increased risk in children with epilepsy
  —slightly increased risk with most other illness
- Specific developmental delay, such as speech and communication difficulty
- Academic failure
- Low self esteem.

The cumulative effect of stress can have a potent negative influence on children. Children who have experienced more than two adverse life events in the recent past are particularly susceptible to developing emotional or behavioural problems. There is evidence that some life stress factors may lie dormant for many years (the sleeper effect) only to have an effect when "awoken" by a related adverse experience. This increased vulnerability to stress may be seen in the abnormal behaviour of some teenagers who have been sexually abused or subjected to other detrimental influences much earlier in their childhood.

Boys are generally more prone to develop psychiatric disorder much as they are more vulnerable to almost every life adversity. The difference in the rate of psychiatric disorders in girls and boys tends to be less pronounced in preschool children. During adolescence, however, girls become more vulnerable, mainly because they have higher rates of emotional disorder. Throughout childhood boys are more likely to experience developmental disorders, behaviour problems, and conduct disorder.

Family and other external risk factors

Family risk factors are especially complex as there are many possible interactions (box 3). Family breakdown is a good example of a process of adverse events and interactions that multiply the risk of psychopathology. Thus, children from a broken home may copy the parental model of unsatisfactory relationships and poor communication, and become increasingly difficult to manage. The child's behaviour is then likely to lead to critical and hostile parental responses that only serve to make the child more disturbed. This results in a prevalence of psychiatric disorder as high as 80% in the first year after divorce. The rate of childhood psychiatric disorder is also raised before and for many years after parental separation. This contrasts with the loss of a parent by death, which gives only a slightly increased risk of psychiatric disorder.

Box 3—Family factors that increase the risk of psychiatric disorder
- Family breakdown
- Maternal mental ill health
- Paternal criminality, alcoholism, psychopathy
- Abuse
- Poverty—whatever the cause
- Overt parental conflict
- Inconsistent, unclear, or critical discipline
- Hostile and rejecting relationships
- Failure to adapt to child's developmental needs
- Death and loss—including loss of friendships.

Maternal, but not paternal, mental illness increases the risk of psychiatric disorder. A child's vulnerability to a depressed mother may be increased during critical periods of development, for example during the time when the mother is bonding to the child in the first few weeks after birth. There is also evidence that some children continue to have problems even after the mother's depression has resolved, suggesting that a process of negative behaviour has been established that becomes difficult to disentangle. Very young children are strongly influenced by the mood of their parents, but as they grow older other factors such as school, peers, and culture have a more powerful effect. Children spend a minimum of some 15 000 hours in school. It is therefore no surprise to find that experiences at school, such as bullying, school organisation, and academic achievement can influence the rate of childhood psychiatric disorder (box 4).

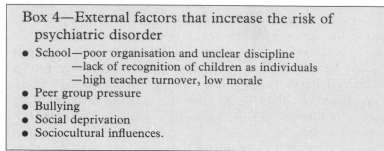

Box 4—External factors that increase the risk of psychiatric disorder
- School—poor organisation and unclear discipline
            —lack of recognition of children as individuals
            —high teacher turnover, low morale
- Peer group pressure
- Bullying
- Social deprivation
- Sociocultural influences.

Protective factors against psychiatric disorders in children

The risk factors outlined above are common to many children and yet only a minority at any one time actually suffer from a formal psychiatric disorder. So why do some children survive and not develop a psychiatric disorder even though they have many adversities stacked up against them? One of the most powerful protective factors of all is a positive self esteem. Self image develops slowly and becomes relatively fixed by 7–8 years of age. It is crucially dependent on how parents and others have responded to the child. The presence of an affectionate and trusting relationship with an adult is therefore also protective. A stable temperament and a good level of intelligence will help a child to adapt to stressful situations and reduce the risk of psychiatric disorder (box 5).

Box 5—Factors that protect against psychiatric disorder
- Positive self image
- Affectionate relationships
- Supportive relationships with adults
- Stable personality
- Having a special skill
- High IQ and academic achievement
- Parents who give high levels of supervision and clear discipline.

Assessment of psychiatric disorder in children

The evaluation of psychiatric disorder in very young children may seem to be inappropriate, as thoughts and feelings are still developing and rapidly changing in this age group. Nevertheless, preschool children do experience strong emotions, which they communicate most expressively with their behaviour and their play. Thus surveillance assessment of young children will have to focus most carefully on how the child behaves in various situations. An additional complicating factor in assessing younger children is that they tend to reflect the moods and attitudes of their main carer. The child–parent relationship and the mental state of the parent therefore forms an important part of the assessment for psychiatric disorder.

Assessing children and their relationships is a complex process in which the observations of parents and teachers must play a major part. Information about the child has to be gathered from as many sources as possible. Even so, a child's disturbance is often situation specific, with reports of problem behaviour in one setting only. Psychiatric disorders that are manifest in one situation only do not necessarily mean that the cause of the problem must also be there: a child may be difficult at home because of academic failure at school or present major problems at school because of abuse at home.

The assessment process must therefore take account of the context in which the problems occur and note how each aetiological factor interacts with the others to generate the problem. It is helpful to start by considering the contribution that the child makes to the development of the disorder and then go on to review the role of the family and finally the influence of school and the outside world, as outlined in boxes 2–5.

Screening for psychiatric disorder

Parents and teachers will always be a major source of information, but as children grow older it becomes increasingly relevant to obtain details from the children themselves. Most children aged under 7–8 years find it difficult to report their own feelings or to give a considered view of how they perceive the world. Nevertheless, it is always worth while directly questioning younger children to see what they have to say, provided that this is put in a developmental context. Accordingly, whatever the age of the child, it is important to use direct observation and questioning of the child, rather than to rely solely on the reports of others.

Questionnaires and rating scales can be used to screen children for psychiatric disorder. These are mostly aimed at parents and teachers, but new scales are now being developed for older children to rate their own symptoms. On the face of it, questionnaires might seem to be the answer to the problem of screening large numbers of children for psychiatric disorder, but caution is required as all scales are subject to error and throw up both false positive and false negative results.

Young children can be assessed on the preschool behaviour questionnaire.[1] School age children can be screened with the Rutter A (parents) and the Rutter B (teachers) scales which measure common emotional and behavioural problems.[2] Both checklists are well established as properly validated and reliable scales. They are short and easy to administer. A longer, but equally well established, schedule is the child behaviour checklist.[3]

Early signs of psychiatric disorder

Adverse temperamental characteristics can be recognised soon after birth and are associated with an appreciable increase in the risk of behaviour problems developing at a later stage. Other qualities, such as the appearance and gender of the child will also play a part in determining parental perceptions and responses. The seeds for future parent–child relationship problems may be sown during this early stage, but it is important not to see these early experiences as fixed and unresponsive to outside influences.

The risk of poor early child care and parent–child relationship problems is increased if the mother has received poor child care herself. A parent who required special schooling for learning difficulties as a child, and very young parents, are also likely to find child care a problem. Fortunately, deficiencies in mothering can be compensated for by a supportive father or other caring adult (box 6).

Although it is vital not to assume that there will inevitably be problems if one or more risk factors are present, careful surveillance should be maintained until it is clear that good progress is being made. Direct observation of parental behaviour with the baby is more reliable than what parents actually say. Surveillance in the first few weeks should therefore focus on parent–child interactions and should particularly note the parental responses

---

Box 6—Factors that make child care more difficult

- Unsupported single parent
- Maternal depression
- Limited intellectual ability (IQ less than 70%)
- Teenage pregnancy
- Poor parental relationship
- Poor parenting experience as a child
- Lack of paternal involvement
- Persistent rejection of the child after the first three months.

---

listed in box 7. Any problem that might be noted in the parent–child relationship at this early stage is not necessarily serious. Most parents will resolve any difficulties within a few months. But this early period is a critical time when support and encouragement for the more vulnerable parents can be especially effective.

Box 7—Checklist for assessing parenting of very young children

- Feeding
- Attending to basic child care tasks
- Playing with and talking to the baby
- Responding to distress and crying
- Protecting from danger
- Showing affection.

The preschool child

The range of emotional and behavioural symptoms is relatively limited in the preschool years. At this stage of rapid maturation any emotional or physical stress will cause obvious regression to more immature behaviour. It is therefore important not to be overimpressed by the apparently dramatic appearance of regressive behaviour during a physical illness, or with emotional distress or excitement. However, the behaviour should return to normal within a period of days or weeks once the stress is removed. A sound knowledge of child development is necessary to put any immaturity in perspective and thus distinguish between generally delayed development, specific developmental delay, and regression.

On starting primary school a child should have reached a reasonable level of social acceptability, and at this stage psychiatric

9

disorders tend to present as immature behaviour. The main areas for psychiatric surveillance in preschool children are shown in box 8.

Box 8—Check list for preschool children

- Feeding and sleeping patterns
- Activity level and concentration
- Bowel and bladder control
- Temper and impulse control
- Separation anxiety
- Responsiveness to social cues
- Ability to communicate basic needs.

Emotional and behavioural disorders in preschool children are relatively non-specific, and the range of normal behaviour is so great that it is often difficult to decide what is abnormal. It is best to adopt a pragmatic approach to diagnosing psychiatric disorder in preschool children, and it may help to pose the simple question: Is the child's reaction "*out of proportion*" to what might normally be expected in the circumstances, and is the child or the carer handicapped as a result?

The school age child

The role of parents and the family in generating psychiatric disorder is crucial in younger children, but as children grow older other factors gradually grow more important and the influence of the school and of other children becomes relatively greater. Surveillance at this stage needs to take into account what is happening at school and events outside the family in addition to the dynamics of the family itself.

Starting school is an important maturational experience. Children are assessed on their own merits in a more critical and detached way than most parents find possible. This may lead to temporary difficulties such as separation problems or disobedience. Appropriate management at school in liaison with the child's home should bring about a rapid resolution, thus distinguishing these transient difficulties from a more serious psychiatric disorder.

Young children are remarkably resilient, but as they grow older and become more self aware they are increasingly influenced by the attitudes of others. By 8 years old most children have a reasonably clear view of themselves and how they compare with other youngsters. At this age, a child can develop a sense of failure and a low self esteem, which will greatly increase the risk of emotional and behavioural problems.

Regression and immature behaviour are relatively more important if they occur in older children. For example, enuresis in children older than 7 or 8 years is likely to result in low self esteem, thereby making the child more vulnerable to failure in other areas of functioning, such as school work. Overactivity is another symptom that has added seriousness when it occurs in school age children. Inattentiveness and distractibility will interfere with learning, which in turn may provoke negative responses from teachers and other children. This can quickly result in a vicious cycle of failure, distress, opting out, and disruptive behaviour.

Surveillance for emotional and behavioural disorders in school age children should include factors that have been considered for younger children, but should also focus on more subtle areas of functioning, such as how the child manages relationships and the child's self perception and ability to control impulses. Academic achievement plays a critical role at this stage, so ability to concentrate and to read and write at an age appropriate level will strongly influence a child's mental state (see box 9).

Box 9—Check list for school age children
- Academic progress, especially ability to read
- Relationships with adults and children
- Self esteem
- Concentration span
- Mood state
- Impulse control.

Symptoms that indicate serious psychopathology

Most psychiatric conditions in childhood are disorders of mental functioning and not illnesses. The distinction being that a disorder is an exaggeration of normal symptoms to the point that they become handicapping—a quantitative difference—and an illness is qualitatively different from normality. Thus most emotional and behavioural symptoms are relatively non-specific, and the presence of a single symptom will give little intimation of the seriousness of the underlying psychopathology. It is the pattern of associated symptoms and the context in which they occur that gives a better indication. However, some symptoms are strongly associated with definite psychiatric disorder, even when they occur in isolation. These symptoms are listed in box 10 and should always be seen as having potentially serious implications, warranting detailed assessment and careful management.

Box 10—Check list of potentially serious symptoms

- Persistent deliberate destructiveness
- Aggression leading to injury
- Deliberate self harm
- Sexual behaviour inappropriate to age
- Fire setting
- Social disinhibition
- Persistent isolation and withdrawal
- Bizarre behaviour
- Hallucinations and delusions.

Symptoms with a particularly poor prognosis

The serious symptoms of mental dysfunction listed in box 10 are indicative of pronounced psychopathology, but do not necessarily mean a poor prognosis if appropriate treatment is provided at an early stage. There are, however, a few specific symptoms of childhood that have a particularly poor long term prognosis. They are listed in box 11.

Box 11—Disorders with a generally poor outlook

- Persistent aggressive behaviour after the age of 6–7 years
- Hyperactivity associated with conduct disorder
- Severe, persistent depressive disorder
- Bizarre behaviour
- Low self esteem associated with being abused
- Persistent truancy, especially from primary school
- Repeated running away or suicidal attempts.

After identification—what then?

A successful identification or surveillance programme will identify many children with psychiatric disorder. Awareness of their distress is only helpful if it leads to positive help and support. The issue of what to do with identified children needs to be agreed and

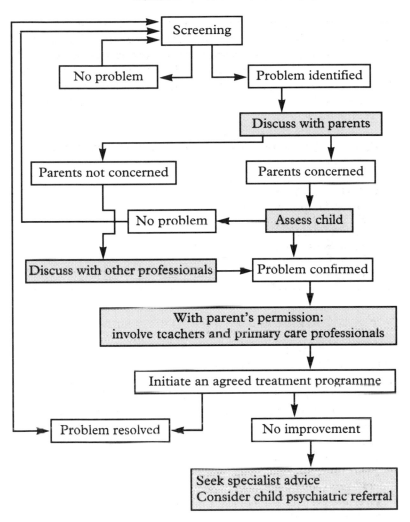

Surveillance of emotional and behavioural problems in children

planned well before any surveillance programme is started. A series of decisions have to be made so that the most seriously disturbed children are provided with appropriate treatment. At the same time, it is necessary to avoid labelling children as being disturbed if the disorder is mild or likely to be transient. The flow chart suggests the decision making steps and responses that can be taken as part of a surveillance process.

13

Conclusions

The identification of mental health problems in children is a complex matter and has to take a wide range of different factors into account. An overall rate for psychiatric disorder of 7–14% can be expected in the general child population. This means that many children will be identified in a surveillance process. However, not all these children will require formal psychiatric assessment and treatment. Many can be helped by their parents and by appropriately skilled professionals. Informal psychiatric advice may be helpful at an early stage before a problem has become firmly established. Close collaboration with colleagues in the child psychiatry service is therefore important.

1 McGuire J, Richman N. 1986. Screening for behaviour problems in nurseries. The reliability and validity of the preschool behavior checklist. *J Child Psychol Psychiatry* 1986;27:7–32.
2 Rutter M, Tizard J, Yule W, Graham P, Whitmore K. Isle of Wight studies 1964–1974. *Psychol Med* 1976;7:313–32.
3 Achenbach TM, Edelbrock C. 1983. *Manual for the child behavior checklist and revised child behavior profile.* Burlington, Vermont: University of Vermont, Dept of Psychiatry, 1983.

Further reading

Graham P. *Child psychiatry: a developmental approach.* Oxford: Oxford University Press, 1991. (An excellent short textbook.)

2. Types of psychiatric treatment

Philip J Graham

The aim of this book is to provide paediatricians and other doctors with information about therapeutic approaches used in departments of child and adolescent psychiatry. Such information can be seen not just as having general educational value. All paediatricians see a high proportion of children with behavioural and emotional disturbances.[12] Only a small proportion are referred—many are not because the child psychiatric resources are inadequate, because parents are not motivated, or because the disturbances, although bothersome, are not serious enough. In all these cases the paediatrician may find it helpful to apply some of the ideas described in this book. This may sound like encouragement of dangerous dabbling. But paediatricians are inevitably forced into situations where they try to help families with disturbed children, and provided that they proceed with caution, are appropriately self critical, and preferably have the opportunity to discuss what they are doing with a mental health professional from time to time, my observations suggest that they can indeed be extremely helpful.

Definitions

Psychiatric treatment covers all therapeutic approaches used for children with emotional and behavioural disturbances.[3] Types of treatment can be divided into *psychological therapies* and *physical therapies*. Psychological therapies include those that primarily aim to uncover underlying conflicts, tensions, and drives of which the child and family members were previously unaware and which are thought to be the covert source of the problem. These insight promoting therapies are termed *psychoanalytic* if clearly derived from the work of early psychoanalysts, especially Sigmund and Anna Freud and Melanie Klein. The term psychoanalytic treatment is usually reserved for quite intensive (three to five times a

15

Box 1—Types of psychiatric treatment

Psychological
   Psychodynamic, psychoanalytic
   Behavioural
   Cognitive behavioural
Physical
   Medication
   Diet.

week) individual treatment, and it is more likely to be termed psychotherapy or psychodynamic therapy if the underlying concepts are the same but treatment is provided on a less frequent basis. Psychological therapies are termed *behavioural* if they aim to alter what the child or family members do by methods that tackle the symptoms directly, or *cognitive behavioural* if they aim to produce behaviour change by altering patterns of thought. However, psychological therapies can also be classified according to the unit (individual, family, group) to which the therapy is applied. Those engaged in family therapy[4] may use psychodynamic or behavioural concepts or a mixture of the two. They may also use

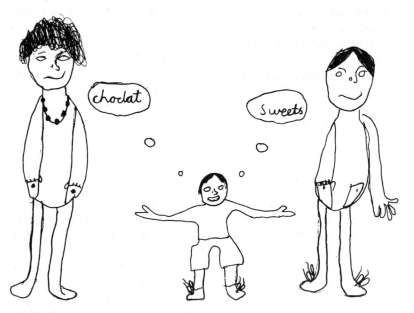

Psychiatric treatment can help children develop more rewarding and trusting relationships with others.

concepts special to family therapists. Thus "systems" therapies are based on the notion that families can be viewed as homoeostatic entities—if you change one part of the system you change the rest.

Physical therapies are less commonly used in children. They include medication, dietary approaches, and electroconvulsive therapy, the last of which is used either extremely rarely or not at all until late adolescence.

Child mental health professionals also provide indirect treatment through consultation without direct clinical contact. *Consultation and liaison work* is carried out especially with paediatricians, social workers, and teachers.

Finally, there are various miscellaneous forms of psychiatric treatment that cannot readily be classified according to the above system. *Hypnosis* aims to allow the child greater control of his or her thoughts and behaviour by means of techniques used while the child is in a state of altered awareness.[56] "Holding therapy", particularly used for children with autism, involves forcible physical contact to overcome the withdrawal such children show.

Not so long ago there was considerable antagonism between psychodynamic therapists and behaviour therapists. Psychodynamic therapists saw behaviourism as superficial tinkering that left the real problems untouched. Behaviourists saw psychodynamic therapists as misguidedly applying an unproved set of theories with little interest in or evidence for success. Such mutual dismissiveness has by no means totally disappeared, but there is distinctly more appreciation of the fact that different forms of treatment can be valuable in different circumstances. The indications and contraindications of different types of treatment will be discussed in later chapters in this book.

Treatment settings and staff

There is a wide variety of settings in which psychiatric treatment is practised. With new purchaser/provider arrangements, the level and variety of services are likely to increase considerably. Community child guidance clinics are now much more commonly termed child and family psychiatric clinics. Child and adolescent departments of child psychiatry may be sited in general hospitals or children's hospitals. Inpatient units usually take either prepubertal children or adolescents, but a minority of larger units admit the entire age range. Some inpatient units also admit a proportion of day patients, and there is a relatively small number of child psychiatric day centres exclusively given over to day patients. Many child mental health staff work in other settings, such as schools for children with emotional and behaviour disorders (EBD schools) and child development clinics.[7]

The professional staff working in any of these centres is likely to be multidisciplinary, and treatment may be delivered by any of the professionals involved. Child psychiatrists have particular skills in formulating clinical problems in which both biological and psychosocial factors are important. They alone among the mental health team will be able to prescribe psychotropic medication. They will probably continue to be the gateholders for inpatient child psychiatric treatment.

As well as child psychiatrists, who are medically trained, there are clinical and educational psychologists (nearly all with teaching experience). Though traditionally psychologists have spent much time systematically testing children, they now spend a much higher proportion of their time devising and sometimes carrying out programmes of treatment. Educational psychologists now also spend much time (some feel too much) in processing statements of special educational need. Especially in London and the south east of England, but much less commonly elsewhere, there are analytically trained child psychotherapists. Although many local authority social workers remain in child and family psychiatric clinics and departments, some have been withdrawn and others are mainly taken up with work in child protection and court work and have little or no time for therapy. Although child psychotherapists have a very specialised training in individual psychoanalytical techniques, they are increasingly becoming involved in liaison work and sometimes family therapy and may work in paediatric outpatient clinics.[8] Child psychiatrists and clinical psychologists are likely to be able to apply a range of therapeutic techniques, including most of those described above. In addition, child psychiatric nurses, although most likely to work in inpatient units or day centres, are now increasingly exercising their skills in the community.

Is child psychiatric treatment effective?

This is nearly, but perhaps not quite as naive a question as "Is paediatric treatment effective?" Although there is an increasing number of studies evaluating effectiveness, well summarised for individual psychotherapy,[9] for family therapy,[10] for behavioural modification,[11] and for medication,[12] the indications and contraindications for particular forms of treatment are still sometimes uncertain. There is, however, good evidence that certain forms of treatment are more suitable for certain conditions than others, as the ensuing chapters in this book will show.

It must be admitted that some practitioners still enthusiastically apply the same form of treatment to virtually all children and families they see, and this is undesirable. For example, the application of individual psychotherapy to the treatment of conduct disorders can be seriously questioned on the basis of existing evidence. Such relatively absolute contraindications can be matched by relatively absolute indications for certain types of treatment. For example, the uses of medication in the more severe forms of hyperkinesia and Tourette's syndrome, of a mixture of individual and family psychotherapy in anorexia nervosa, and of behavioural treatment in nocturnal enuresis and monosymptomatic phobias are well established. However, for a variety of other common disorders such as anxiety and depressive states, and for conduct disorders, non-specific factors such as the enthusiasm of the therapist or therapeutic team are probably of greater importance than the specific type of treatment used. Paediatricians in training who find themselves working with psychiatrists and psychologists with different therapeutic orientations may be confused, but should find that they can learn much that is of value from observing the application of different approaches to similar problems.[13] In particular, they may benefit as much from observing how child mental health professionals can clarify the nature of a problem, helping the family and themselves to see the problem in a different way, as from observing specific treatment interventions.

As the classification systems used in child psychiatry become more refined, there will probably be increasing precision in our application of particular types of treatment. In the meantime, it would be highly desirable for evaluative studies to include not only scientifically valid controlled trials but also measures of consumer satisfaction. With increasing dependence on their "customers", among whom they must certainly count paediatricians, child mental health professionals will be increasingly sensitive to what their clients think of their interventions.

> ## Box 2—Indications for referral to a child psychiatric service (if available)
>
> 1 Emotional or behaviour problems unresponsive to first line counselling
> 2 Problematic child protection cases
> 3 Difficult diagnostic problems (no obvious organic cause).

Indications for referral

Referral to a child psychiatrist or a child mental health service is not really a problematic issue for paediatricians who work closely with their psychiatric colleagues, see them at regular weekly psychosocial meetings and, at least occasionally, at lunch, and who have the opportunity to see which children and families seem to benefit and which do not. For those with less close contacts, some guidelines may be helpful.[14] Children who are appreciably functionally disabled by persistent problems that either have no organic basis or an insufficient organic explanation need referral, and the earlier they are referred the better. Some paediatricians have found it helpful to use routinely a screening questionnaire to identify children at risk for psychosocial problems (see also chapter 1).[15] When it is clear from the outset that children presenting with difficult diagnostic problems probably have a non-organic explanation for symptoms, the children should be referred early on— preferably while the investigatory stage is under way—so that when all investigations are proved negative the child psychiatric department is not used as a last resort or "dustbin" department, but the child psychiatrist is seen as someone who has been involved from the start. In the occasional child who turns out to have a rare abdominal tumour or degenerative brain disorder to explain abdominal pains or headaches, the early involvement of a psychiatrist need not antagonise parents if it has been made clear at the outset that the diagnostic process may indeed show an organic cause for symptoms. Problematic child protection cases would also benefit from discussion with a psychiatrist, though in many cases direct clinical psychiatric contact will not be indicated.

Of course, probably only a minority of paediatricians are able to refer to psychiatrists as much as they would wish. Paediatricians who press energetically for an increase in their psychiatric service will usually obtain a better service within a reasonable period of time. One hopeful sign for the future is the gradual emergence of a stronger clinical child psychology service, sometimes, as occurs more frequently in the US,[16] working in close partnership with paediatricians. This will not only be increasingly helpful to paediatricians, but will allow child psychiatrists to concentrate more on hospital and community health work for which their medical and psychiatric training has specifically equipped them.

1 Costello EJ, Edelbrock C, Costello AJ, Dulcan MK, Burns BJ, Brent D. Psychopathology in pediatric primary care: the new hidden morbidity. *Pediatrics* 1988;**82**:415–24.

2 Garralda ME, Bailey D. Psychiatric disorders in general paediatric referrals. *Arch Dis Child* 1989;**64**:1727–33.

3 Graham P. *Child psychiatry: a developmental approach.* 2nd Ed. Oxford: Oxford University Press, 1991.

4 Lask B. Family therapy. *BMJ* 1987;**294**:203–4.

5 Olness K. Hypnotherapy in children. *Postgrad Med* 1986;**79**:95–105.

6 Sokel B, Lansdown R, Kent A. The development of a hypnotherapy service for children. *Child Care Health Dev* 1990;**16**:227–33.

7 Evered CJ, Hill PD, Hall PM, Hollins SC. Liaison psychiatry in a child development clinic. *Arch Dis Child* 1989;**64**:745–8.

8 Vas Dias S, McKenzie SA. Paediatric psychotherapy: a service in a general outpatient clinic. *Arch Dis Child* 1992;**67**:132–4.

9 Barrnett RJ, Docherty JP, Frommelt GM. A review of psychotherapy research since 1963. *J Am Acad Child Adolesc Psychiatry* 1991;**30**:1–14.

10 Markus E, Lange A, Pettigrew TF. Effectiveness of family therapy—a meta-analysis. *Journal of Family Therapy* 1990;**12**:205–21.

11 Werry JS, Wollersheim JP. Behaviour therapy with children and adolescents: a twenty-year overview. *J Am Acad Child Adolesc Psychiatry* 1989;**28**:1–18.

12 Campbell M, Spencer EK. Psychopharmacology in child and adolescent psychiatry: a review of the past five years. *J Am Acad Child Adolesc Psychiatry* 1988;**27**:269–79.

13 Graham P, Jenkins S. Training of paediatricians for psychosocial aspects of their work. *Arch Dis Child* 1985;**60**:777–80.

14 Graham P. Paediatric referral to a child psychiatrist. *Arch Dis Child* 1984;**59**:1103–5.

15 Jellinek M, Murphy JM, Burns B. Brief psychosocial screening in out-patient pediatric practice. *J Pediatr* 1986;**109**:371–8.

16 Kannoy KW, Schroeder CS. Suggestions to parents about common behavior problems in a pediatric primary care office: 5 years of follow-up. *J Pediatr Psychol* 1985;**10**:15–30.

PART II
SPECIFIC TYPES
OF TREATMENT

3. Individual psychotherapy

Judith Trowell

Definition

Individual psychodynamic psychotherapy involves one to one treatment using verbal and play techniques. The treatment is based on working with the patient in the here and now—that is, on the relationship that develops between the patient and the therapist. Links are constantly made from this to past experiences and current external relationships.

The difficulties of a child or young person with a psychiatric disorder are understood as arising from internal and external conflicts and trauma. How these are dealt with using psychodynamic theories depends on early experiences of significant relationships modified by subsequent relationships and also on the stage the patient has reached in his or her developmental pathway. The external conflicts and traumas resonate with internal unconscious conflicts and traumas, and hence can exacerbate the patients' inability to manage their current difficulties. Thus the behaviour and pattern of relationships can become "stuck", often repeating previous distressing or unhelpful or destructive patterns. Anna Freud described the developmental pathways and defences as she saw them;[1] Melanie Klein described her view of development and the normal and abnormal processes she understood from her work with severely disturbed and damaged children.[2] Winnicott, in his therapeutic work alongside his paediatric work and psychosocial liaison, made his particular contribution in understanding childhood distress and what was required for healthy mental and physical development.[3] Bowlby's attachment theory describes the importance of early relationships as a focus for current relationships, and his concept of a secure base can be helpful in providing a secure treatment setting where dysfunctional relationships can be re-enacted.[4]

Individual psychotherapy can be used with children from about 18 months to 2 years of age and through childhood and adolescence. Before 18 months parent–child psychotherapy is used instead, in which the therapist works with the parent and child or with the child with the help of the parent.

The importance of the setting

One of the features of individual treatment is to try and provide a consistent, regular, reliable setting for the treatment. This means wherever possible making the treatment sessions on the same day, at the same time, in the same room, and with the same play equipment and toys available. This may be in a child and family mental health clinic or in a department of child psychiatry or department of psychological medicine. Children can also be seen at school, whether primary, secondary, or a special school, if a room can be made available. Children and young people can also be seen in hospital on a paediatric ward, a child psychiatry ward, an adolescent unit, or a day unit. The child or young person does need some privacy and if at all possible some physical space without too many intrusions such as telephone calls or people coming in and out.

Play materials provided vary with age, and preschool children generally have crayons, paper, plasticine, plastic small farm and wild animals, simple plastic figures, cars, and pipe cleaner dolls. Primary schoolchildren are more inclined to use paper, scissors, glue, felt tip pens, cars, a ball, and string as well as plasticine, the animals, and figures. Secondary schoolchildren may prefer to talk, although many of them like to draw or write.

Which children and young people can benefit?

Children and young people can become distressed, confused, and depressed by life's adversities. Some of them may have particularly difficult circumstances and some may be vulnerable children. If a child or young person becomes stuck and unable to resolve the difficulties with the help of the usual resources— parents, teachers, family friends, their general practitioner, or a counsellor in school—they may benefit from treatment.

Other children and young people may be much more floridly troubled and have very worrying or disturbed behaviour that is

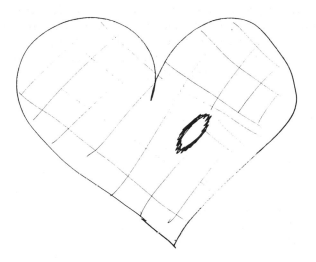

Children and young people can become distressed, confused, and depressed by life's adversities. This picture was drawn by a child aged 8 in contested adoption. "All my love is for John and Mary (prospective adopters), but they'll always be a little bit in the middle for my born-to Mum."

dangerous to themselves or others. Very disturbed children with psychotic features can respond well to treatment, children with developmental delay can also improve considerably. I would like to suggest nine categories of problems for which individual psychotherapy should be considered.[5]

(1) Family breakdown and reconstituted families. Some children may be caught between warring parents or in a very difficult new family situation. Individual treatment, perhaps with family therapy, can help the children sort out their own feelings and reactions to the emotional turmoil.[6]

(2) Life events such as bereavement loss of a parent or a sibling, physical or mental handicap in a sibling, or suicide of a parent or sibling can leave many children and young people confused and bewildered and they can benefit from individual treatment.[78]

(3) A child or young person with chronic physical or mental handicap may have serious emotional difficulties and conflicts that can prevent them from being able to use what mental or physical capacities they do have. Individual treatment can liberate them to enable them to develop in ways that they can and to enable them to find some satisfaction in the relationships they can develop.

27

Adolescents may need particular help with their sexual feelings, needs, and wishes.[9][10]

(4) Paediatric liaison. Children and young people with acute or chronic conditions on the hospital ward may not be able to maximise their use of the skilled care they receive because of emotional difficulties and distress. Individual treatment can help them make sense of their experiences and their feelings so that they can respond more positively to those around, staff, and parents.[11]

(5) Many children who have been abused have emotional sequelae. Emotional abuse can profoundly traumatise the child. Physical abuse, neglect, and sexual abuse usually involve considerable emotional abuse. Children's sense of self, self esteem, awareness of boundaries (that is, a sense of themselves as separate people with emotional space between self and other), ability to think their own thoughts, have their own feelings, own their own bodies, have all been attacked. Some of these children need individual treatment urgently. Other abused children, once in a safe place, want to settle into a normal life and do not want at this time to talk about the abuse. Many of these children need help later, for example, a sexually abused 7 year old girl may become very troubled at puberty, when she has a boyfriend, marries, becomes pregnant, or has a baby. She may need individual treatment at any or all of these transitions.[12-15]

(6) Children and young people with psychosomatic conditions for which there may be emotional factors, such as asthma, diabetes, or eczema, can benefit from psychotherapy. There are also children and young people with quite severe problems such as abdominal pain to non-organic paralyses, which lead to frequent hospital admissions, who can experience considerable improvement with psychotherapy.[16][17]

(7) Developmental delay can be generalised or specific. Children with overall delay often have emotional difficulties with autistic or psychotic features. Individual psychotherapy for these children is very specialised and the technique has needed modification, but some children can be helped to move forward.

Children with specific delays, language or numeracy delay, may have emotional factors that can be released. Children who are enuretic or encopretic can benefit, although many of them are difficult to help.[18-21]

(8) Children in transition in foster families or in adoptive families often have had very difficult experiences and are unable to use the new relationships because of the emotional pain, rage, and

hurt confusion locked inside them. Individual psychotherapy can free them to engage appropriately with their new carers and can help avoid frequent breakdown of placements.[22][23]

(9) Adolescents have particular transitions and emotional turmoils. Because they are so volatile and fluctuating they can often make good use of a small number of sessions to make sense of their distress or confusion. Overdoses, anorexia nervosa, substance abuse, teenage pregnancy, leaving home, and moving to work or further education, can all lead to unresolvable difficulties. Some of the young people may respond to individual treatment but unlike young children they need to consent and bring themselves so the number taking advantage of this treatment is limited.[24][25]

Lush 1991

Box 1—Some indications for individual psychodynamic psychotherapy

Children who have difficulties in coping with distress caused by the following life adversities:

- Family breakdown
- Bereavement or illness in the family
- Chronic physical/mental handicap
- Physical illness
- Abuse, emotional/sexual/physical
- Somatisation of distress
- Developmental delays
- In transition—fostering/adoption
- Adolescent turmoil.

Therapists and treatment

Individual psychotherapy is available from child and adolescent psychotherapists and child and adolescent psychiatrists if they have specialised in this therapeutic method. Child psychotherapists are generally psychologists, social workers, or teachers who have undertaken a postgraduate training.

Educational therapists are teachers who have undertaken further training in applying this treatment in the school setting to children with learning difficulties. Play therapists, nurses, and occupational therapists use some of the skills either with regular supervision by a therapist or after a postqualification course in therapeutic communication with children.

Treatment can be brief, for example five sessions offered to an adolescent, or focused to work on a particular problem such as a bereavement or an inpatient admission. It can vary in frequency: generally it is once a week but for a very small number of children or adolescents who are very troubled it can be twice or three times a week. Very rarely indeed a child might be seen four or five times a week. Treatment may be time limited or may be open ended and reviewed at regular intervals and decisions on how to proceed then agreed.

Treatment is terminated when the child or young person ceases to be preoccupied with their conflicts or difficulties and better able to fulfil their potential and establish satisfying relationships. Improvement can continue for up to two years after treatment so the precise moment when to stop is still a matter of clinical judgment. Young people often vote with their feet and they decide when treatment will cease. Young children stop coming because the carer finds regular attendance difficult or continue coming for too long because the parents long to have their child "transformed". The work then has to shift into helping parents accept their child's condition.

For treatment to be sustained, most carers need regular discussion time with professional members of the clinical team to feel part of and involved in the treatment and to share their concerns. Children and adolescents recover more quickly and in general recovery is consolidated faster if the carers are actively involved with a worker exploring their part in the interactional problems and helping them think about how they can help their child.

Box 2—Individual psychodynamic psychotherapy: treatment strategies

- Listening, non-directiveness, insight-promoting interpretations
- Regular, predictable sessions of predetermined duration in a consistent setting
- Use of play and drawing materials
- Development of a therapeutic relationship with the therapist, re-enactment of dysfunctional relationships, exploration and understanding of these patterns, followed by the opportunity to try alternative means of dealing with anxiety, conflict, and relationships
- Opportunity to review and reflect on the available choices or options, considering what are external factors and what are internal and hence what can and cannot be changed internally and externally.

Why psychotherapy can help children cope with life stresses

It used to be thought that children "grow out" of emotional difficulties even if conduct disorders were predictors of problems in adult life. It is now recognised that children and young people with emotional disorders or mixed emotional and conduct disorders go on to have emotional and relationship problems in adult life. Therapeutic interventions can change this.[26]

Children and young people are generally resilient, many of them cope and can use resources available, for example a telephone help line, a professional, a teacher, their general practitioner, someone in the family or extended family, a friend, or a neighbour. But many pay a price in later life, children in divorcing families are more likely to divorce themselves, sexually abused children have relationship difficulties and mental health problems. Children unable to learn because of emotional problems do not achieve and can have frustrated and unsatisfying lives.

It is not always the obvious life events that cause the problem, but whether the child has internal emotional strength from good enough parenting—that is, whether the current difficulty comes on top of pre-existing vulnerability. It does seem increasingly clear that without help troubled children become troubled adults in dysfunctional families. Of course, if a child is subject to a particular stress or a disaster then this may adversely affect the most robust of children and leave them with a post-traumatic stress disorder.[27]

Effects of treatment

Outcome studies are sparse and more are currently being undertaken. Previous studies tended to be global and now that projects are looking at which treatment for which problem with which child and which therapist, the benefits are emerging, showing that therapeutic interventions do bring immediate and long term benefits to children with a wide range of difficulties.

Can psychotherapy be practised by paediatricians?

Many paediatricians are very effective at communicating with children about their feelings. Winnicott in his therapeutic consultations with children showed how effective these contacts can be.[31]

Some paediatricians undertake a course on therapeutic communication with children, but for them to provide regular treatment for some of the very troubled children would not make sense. A non-medical therapist would more appropriately provide this intervention in consultation with the child and adolescent psychiatrist.

Specialised training is needed

Individual psychotherapy requires assessment skills and communication skills. But it also requires enormous reserves of understanding, compassion, firmness, resilience, humour, courage, perseverance, and awareness of oneself and one's own competence, authority, and appropriate professional behaviour. To achieve this a very thorough in depth training is required.

When children and young people confide in a therapist they can be very vulnerable, their feelings and their pain make them easily open to exploitation, and therapists who lack personal awareness may all too easily use the child or young person to meet their own emotional needs. An essential aspect of any training is that therapists must be aware of their own experiences and how their own lives have affected them, so that they know when they might respond inappropriately.

Contraindications to treatment

If a child or young person is experiencing a particular external reality—moving to another area, transferring to boarding school, about to take GCSE exams—it is not appropriate to embark on an intense piece of work. Opening up very painful, distressing areas when there is no time to work them through or when the child or young person must go outside and function can be damaging. A therapeutic consultation would be the right way to proceed in such a situation.

There are also dangers if therapists find themselves out of their depth and unable to cope with a child's rage, pain, distress, or desperate need for affection.

To avoid behaving inappropriately the therapist needs to be very clear about what is treatment and what is parenting. Suicidal young people or children experiencing abuse all need to be placed somewhere safe and be adequately parented or cared for; therapy can never replace parenting or provide monitoring. In cases that involve physical illness, acute or chronic, it is important to work with the general practitioner or paediatrician.

Services across the United Kingdom

In the past, the availability of skilled individual psychodynamic psychotherapy in the UK was restricted to the London area. However, in the past 10 years there have been attempts to move out of London and there has been a blossoming of interest around the country. Training centres now exist in Edinburgh, Leeds, and Birmingham and courses are run in Bristol, Cardiff, Manchester, Liverpool, Newcastle, Oxford, and Cambridge. Trainees are also travelling from other cities to centres so that there are more services available. Much development is still necessary, however, before adequate cover of even one centre per region is possible. Child and adolescent psychotherapists and psychiatrists with a special interest in children and adolescents are committed to developing this specialty.[32]

1 Freud A. *Normality and pathology in childhood*. New York: International Universities Press, 1965.
2 Klein M. *The psychoanalysis of children*. London: Hogarth Press, 1975.
3 Winnicott DW. *Collected papers. Through paediatrics to psychoanalysis*. London: Tavistock, 1958.
4 Bowlby J. *Making and breaking of affectional bonds*. London: Tavistock, 1979.
5 Trowell J. The relevance of current clinical practice in child psychotherapy to child psychiatry. *Psychoanalytic Psychotherapy in the NHS* 1985;1:1–12.
6 Wallerstein J, Blakeslee S. *Second chances. Men, women and children a decade after divorce*. London: Bantam Press, 1989.
7 Bowlby J. *Attachment and loss. Vol 3. Loss*. London: Hogarth Press, 1980.
8 McDougall J. The dead father. *Int J Psychoanal* 1989;70:205–19.
9 Sinason V. Secondary mental handicap and its relationship to trauma. *Psychoanalytic Psychotherapy in the NHS* 1986;2:131–54.
10 Judd D. *Giving sorrow words: working with a dying child*. London: Free Association Books, 1990.
11 Sinason V, Gluckman C. Work with children with an illness or disability. *Journal of Child Psychotherapy* 1990;16:1–111 (special edition).
12 Trowell J. Physical abuse of children. Some consideration when seen from a dynamic perspective. *Psychoanalytic Psychotherapy in the NHS* 1986;2:63–73.
13 Kraemer S. Splitting and stupidity in child sexual abuse. *Psychoanalytic Psychotherapy in the NHS* 1988;3:247–57.
14 Sinason V. Spitting, swallowing, sickening and stupefying the effects of sexual abuse on the child. *Psychoanalytic Psychotherapy in the NHS* 1988;3:1–97.
15 Trowell J. Listening to, talking to and understanding children—reality, imagination, dreams and fantasy. In: Bannister A, Barrett K, Shearer E, eds. *Listening to children*. Essex: Longman for the National Society for the Prevention of Cruelty to Children, 1990.
16 Moran G, Fonagy P. Psychoanalysis and diabetic control: a single case study. *Br J Med Psychol* 1987;60:357–72.

17 Bolton A, Cohen P. Escape with honour: the need for face saving. *Bulletin of the Anna Freud Centre* 1986;**9**:19–34.
18 Spensley S. Cognitive deficient, mindlessness and psychotic depression. *Journal of Child Psychotherapy* 1985;**2**:33–50.
19 Tustin F. *The protective shell in children.* London: Karnac Books, 1990.
20 Tustin F. *Autism and childhood psychoses.* London: Hogarth Press, 1972.
21 Daws D, Boston M. *The child psychotherapist and problems of young people.* London: Karnac Books, 1988.
22 Boston M, Szur R. *Psychotherapy with severely depressed children.* London: Routledge Kegan Paul, 1983.
23 Lush D, Boston M, Grainger E. Evaluating psychoanalytic psychotherapy with children: therapists' assessments and predictions. *Psychoanalytic Psychotherapy in the NHS* 1991;**5**:191–234.
24 Copley B, Forryan B. *Therapeutic work with children and young people.* London: Robert Royce, 1987.
25 Laufer M, Laufer E. *Developmental breakdown and psychoanalytic treatment in adolescence.* Yale: Yale University Press, 1989.
26 Rutter M. Services for children with emotional disorders, needs, accomplishments and future developments. *National Association for Child and Family Mental Health Newsletter.* London: National Association for Child and Family Mental Health, 1991;Oct: 1–5.
27 Pynoos R, Nader K. *Mental health disturbances in children exposed to disaster. Prevention and intervention strategies.* American Academy of Child and Adolescent Psychiatry Prevention Project, 1989/90.
28 Kolvin I, Garside RF, Nicol AT, Macmillan A, Wolstenholme E, Leitch IM. *Health starts here—the maladjusted child in the ordinary school.* London: Tavistock, 1981.
29 Kolvin I, Macmillan A, Nicol AR, Wrate RM. Psychotherapy is effective. *J R Soc Med* 1988;**81**:261–6.
30 Barnett RJ, Docherty JP, Frommelt SM. A review of child psychotherapy research since 1963. *J Am Acad Child Adolesc Psychiatry* 1991;**30**:1–14.
31 Winnicott DW. *Therapeutic consultations in child psychiatry.* London: Hogarth Press, 1971.
32 Trowell J, chair. Working party on the development of child psychotherapy services in the UK. Child and adolescent psychiatry specialist section. *Psychiatric Bulletin* 1991;**15**:47–55.

4. Counselling parents in child behaviour therapy

The development of child behaviour therapy

During the past 21 years the field of behaviour therapy with children has expanded considerably. Ollendick cites a 1968 report by Gelfand and Hartman in which only 70 studies relating to child and adolescent behaviour therapy could be found in the literature.[1] By 1981 this figure had expanded to 1000. This growth has continued and so much so that it is now difficult for the practising clinician to keep abreast of developments within the now extensive literature.

In the late 1960s behaviour therapy was characterised by two main approaches. Direct from the principles of operant conditioning, reinforcement procedures were developed for increasing and decreasing behaviour and these found favour mostly in the fields of mental handicap and conduct disorders. The other approach derived its strategies from classic or respondent conditioning and, in the main, included desensitisation techniques and these were used most often to treat children with phobic and emotional disorders.

In the 1970s interest in imitation learning expanded the behaviour therapist's repertoire through the development of a new set of procedures collectively referred to as "social skills training". Finally, the late 1970s and 1980s saw the development of a set of techniques deriving from an interest in cognitive processes. Included among these are self control techniques, self instructional training, coping and problem solving strategies, and approaches for the reversal of dysfunctional thinking. Though these latter procedures have seen use with wide groups of child problems, they have not, as yet, been satisfactorily validated in their use with overt clinical disorders.

One thread running right through the development of child

behaviour therapy has been the idea that therapists, rather than treating the problems exhibited by children, should educate the parents into this role. Inherently, this makes good sense as it is the parents who have the maximum "therapeutic" contact with their children. The approach, which is often referred to as "parent training" and is the subject of this chapter, has enjoyed enormous success and attention, and especially so in the fields of conduct disorder and mental handicap. Traditionally, hallmarks of this approach include: (a) careful family assessment through interviews and observations of parent–child interactions; (b) training parents to monitor and track child behaviour; (c) educating parents in reinforcement principles and a range of allied techniques, such as praising and ignoring (differential attention), simple punishment procedures such as time out from positive reinforcement, methods for establishing agreements between children and parents (contingency contracting), and how to employ star, point, or simple monetary systems for dealing with day to day problems with routine activities; and, finally (d) teaching parents to generalise their successes across behaviours and over time. In this chapter I examine some of the issues relevant to each of these steps but, in particular, discuss aspects pertinent to busy clinicians in routine practice.

When consulted about child behaviour problems, such as tantrums, sleep difficulties, disobedience, and aggressiveness, we are often tempted to jump quickly to advice about firm, consistent management. However, between complaint and successful resolution, several aspects of our approach will influence the likelihood of success. Firstly, our methods of assessment and consequent understanding of the individuals, interactions, and developmental issues may suggest factors other than the behaviour itself, which also require therapeutic attention. Secondly, as therapists, the way in which we interact with the family will in many instances influence the treatment outcome. Thirdly, the manner in which treatment techniques are imparted will affect their utilisation, and finally, experience in the sorts of "road blocks" that may hinder treatment progress will be important. Some aspects of each of these issues are discussed below.

Assessment of child behaviour problems

A basic prerequisite to any treatment advice is an understanding of the behavioural problems, their antecedents, and consequences.

BEHAVIOURAL ANTECEDENTS

Traditionally, people training parents in behavioural therapy techniques have concerned themselves with what is observable, and through this have shown several immediate and frequently occurring problem antecedents. These include vague instructions by parents, frequently repeated instructions, inconsistency in approach to the behaviour, failure to attend to prosocial behaviour, and excessive attention to disruptive behaviour typified by escalating anger and aggression.[2] The consequences for treatment obviously include teaching the parent to observe more accurately, issue clearer and fewer instructions, and to act earlier and more efficiently. However, this focus on immediate antecedents is often only part of the story.

The immediate interaction between parent and child is influenced by a wide range of events, including other interactions, the effects of family and environmental stressors, and the attitudes and beliefs that parents hold about child behaviour. Failure to attend to these will at worst result in unsuccessful treatment.

Dealing with associated family problems

Marital problems may lead to serious disagreements about child management, less time for the child, and impose additional stress on the child.[3] In the face of open conflict, child management is ill advised until such difficulties are resolved or resolving. Perhaps though, in dysfunctional marriages characterised by apathy and lack of interest, advice to one parent may have beneficial effects. Problems between parents may also be expressed in more covert ways. For instance, the child who sleeps with a parent may serve to mask parental sexual difficulties. One way to test such a hypothesis is to question parents about the consequences for them of successful child problem management.

Other family interactional influences may present more subtly, and only became appreciated through careful investigation. Grandparents, for instance, may criticise and undermine parental efforts. This can often be managed either by appropriate parental assertion, ignoring, or at worst by grandparent exclusion. Finally, siblings not perceived as problematic nevertheless often exhibit some problems and therefore may require to be included in treatment.[2] More subtly, if labelled "good", such children may, in maintaining their relative position, persist in covertly provoking the child labelled "bad". In such cases, if intersibling fighting is problematic, then parents may be best advised to ignore fighting to avoid being dragged into a "good"/"bad" labelling game.

Families may be exposed to a range of stressors that have detrimental effects on child rearing. It has been established that in the year or so after parental separation, mothers may have management difficulties especially with their sons.[4] Here, rather than focusing intervention on child management, it may be far more appropriate to support and advise the mother with regard to the enormous adjustment she is having to make. Other stresses, such as parental depression, illness, or child illness, also require appropriate consideration before child management advice is contemplated.

An inquiry into parent day to day coping may reveal ways in which child difficulties can indirectly be alleviated. At the simplest level for instance, adjustments in parents' daily timetable can create more space and thus reduce stress in areas of child management. For example, in one of my cases, a young mother habitually attempted to dress three young children, make breakfast, get them out to school, and complete some household tasks—all in the space of one hour. In situations where organisation is more chaotic, then various problem solving and coping skills strategies may be required.

Multiproblem families pose the greatest challenge for parent trainers. Not only are they multistressed but also they often exhibit a broad range of poor coping skills. Also, it is often assumed that they are deficient in parenting skills, but this is not usually the complete story. Research has shown that these parents can "learn" and successfully use behavioural management techniques, but unfortunately such improvements are often not maintained.[5] It would appear that their problems lie more within dysfunctional attributions and expectations about their children and their life circumstances. In any case, efforts to improve child management in such families will at least require prolonged and diverse treatment.

The importance of parental attitudes

In the early days of parent training an implicit assumption that attitude change would follow behaviour change existed. This was a naive generalisation. At initial interviews, one is often struck by the strength of parental belief statements such as, "I've tried everything and nothing works", "He's just like his father", "He doesn't learn", etc. No doubt, in milder cases, direct behavioural

```
┌─────────────────────────────────────────────┐
│  Influential distant events                  │
│  ● Past failure in child management          │
│  ● Parent depression                         │
│  ● Marital problems                          │
│  ● Lack of social support                    │
│  ● Interfering relatives                     │
│  ● Other major life stressors                │
│  ● Major child health or development         │
│      worries.                                │
└─────────────────────────────────────────────┘
                      ↓
┌─────────────────────────────────────────────┐
│  Parent thoughts                             │
│  ● Nothing works                             │
│  ● He is just like his father               │
│  ● He just does not learn                    │
│  ● I feel so bad when he is upset           │
│  ● I am so busy that I cannot manage this.   │
└─────────────────────────────────────────────┘
                      ↓
┌─────────────────────────────────────────────┐
│  Parent behaviours                           │
│  ● Inconsistent instructions                 │
│  ● Vague instructions                        │
│  ● Ignoring prosocial behaviour              │
│  ● Anger                                     │
│  ● Apathy.                                   │
└─────────────────────────────────────────────┘
                      ↓
┌─────────────────────────────────────────────┐
│  Observed parent–child interaction           │
└─────────────────────────────────────────────┘
```

Some events that may influence quality of parent–child interaction

advice with successful application may extinguish these beliefs. However, in more difficult cases the belief may hinder progress from the beginning.

Take for example, a mother who feels that nothing works, thinks she is a bad parent, and sees her child as failing to learn, and consider how she approaches her child when trying to get him or her to bed. She is likely to feel fed up or angry, or both, and in consequence her approaches to the child will often convey a lack of belief in her own management ability. Frequent failure will re-inforce such dysfunctional beliefs and perhaps also lead to incon-sistency of effort and rule application. Also, other adults may reinforce the beliefs either by taking over the management or, more directly, by criticising the mother. If the therapist is to avoid failure, then some preliminary work with dysfunctional beliefs will often be necessary.

Basically, such preliminary work will involve identifying the beliefs, teaching the parent to monitor them, then learning to examine them according to reality and finally, in consequence, learning to establish more appropriate ones in their place. For example, if the parent considers that "nothing works" then an in depth examination of behavioural incidents to which this is linked is required. Often this will show that what was thought not to work, was not in the first instance applied appropriately. Equally, other behavioural incidents will illustrate that the techniques appropriately applied did work. In cases where dysfunctional thinking is intense and associated with pronounced emotional distress, treatment lasting many sessions may be required. First the dysfunctional thinking will need modifying, next relaxation training and coping strategies may be required for the emotional components, and finally problem solving approaches may be advocated in order to substitute more appropriate and constructive thinking. Such approaches have shown some promise in several difficult topics, such as child abuse.[6]

When severe child behaviour problems, parent dysfunctional thinking, and emotional problems coexist, then it is likely that family rules governing child behaviour may become loose and inconsistently applied. It is of course difficult to track behaviour when the general rules are unclear. As already hinted, it is therefore important in early therapy to spend time discussing rules. For instance, what are the absolute "don'ts" (for example, no throwing things around, no verbal abuse to parents, etc), what behaviour is expected at mealtimes, homework times, and so on.

Parental expectations of child behaviour

One very important facet of parent thinking centres on expecta-tions about child behaviour. Are the expectations of the child, given his or her particular developmental level, appropriate? The child abuse literature frequently refers to the inappropriate expectations that such parents have of their children.[7] For instance, they may expect the child to exhibit high levels of self control at very young ages, or they might expect their baby to respond exclusively to them without being able to appreciate the need for interactional sensitivity and flexibility. Some years ago I treated an 18 month old child who presented with a six month history of persistent crying. As I am behaviourally orientated, I sought an interactional understanding of the problem in terms of attention versus non-attention. Within this framework the results of a prolonged observation failed to produce answers. However, when concepts such as maternal sensitivity to the child were considered, the nature of the problem became clear. Observation showed that the mother was attending to the child indiscriminately in the sense that she failed to respond to social cues emitted by the child. Some simple parent coaching on such issues produced a dramatic resolution within 24 hours! Thus behavioural assessments in general are incomplete unless the parents' complaints of the child behaviour are seen within the context of normal child development. In some cases then, it may be the parents' expectations that require modification and not the child's behaviour.

Expectations from treatment

An early exploration of parent expectati about the future is also often useful. U expect from the treatment may yield u motivation. Generally, parents pushed agencies may view therapy negatively ai this can be addressed early on, then it about a more positive attitude to therap future may be beneficial in two ways. Fii happen if the problems persist may help tion to attempt change now. Secondl consequences of positive change for the only help motivation but may also sugg might consolidate change. For instance, given positive changes, what will you and your child be able to do in the future that you can't do now?

DEFINING THE PROBLEM BEHAVIOUR

Ask several people to define what they mean by child tantrums, and you will find that the definitions vary considerably from person to person. Such a simple test clearly illustrates the importance of gathering very specific information about the occurrence of the problem behaviour, its frequency, and where it occurs. This becomes even more important when parental complaints are vague. For instance, with complaints such as, "she is anxious", one would want clear episodic data about what she does, says, and what emotions are expressed. Information of this type may show that the parents' concerns about the problem are justified, or that their perception of the behaviour is in some way erroneous. For instance, depressed parents often perceive child behaviour as more problematic than it is,[8] or multistressed parents may exhibit inappropriately high standards when making judgments about child behaviour.[7] Clearly, such findings have consequences for the choice of treatment focus. In other instances information may show that the parents have not actually observed the problem of interest, and typical examples of this include intersibling fighting as already discussed. Finally, accurate descriptions of the behaviour will, where appropriate, help the therapist to decide what opposite prosocial behaviour might later be reinforced.

BEHAVIOURAL CONSEQUENCES

Knowledge of the consequences of problem behaviour will obviously increase our understanding about why the problems persist. Interest in consequences will, in most instances, focus on exactly what they are, how frequently they occur, how appropriate they are, and how consistently they are applied. Spreading the inquiry into common positive and negative consequent behaviour employed by the parent will also hint at which may, with or without modification, be utilised later. Finally, information on the relative frequency of negative or positive consequences will be important as this too may require later therapeutic consideration. To illustate: research in families with aggressive children has shown that often parents use more negative than positive consequences.[2]

Previous reference has been made to the parental belief that nothing works. In such cases, careful inquiry into what rewards and punishments they consider don't work may actually show that these techniques (as the parents see them) have paradoxical effects. In other words, when the smack is applied the child behaviour worsens, or when the parent praises, the appropriate behaviour decreases. Clearly, in these cases the techniques are not being employed at sufficient intensity or their timing is inappropriate. In treatment, appropriate corrections or other consequences will need to be found.

There is a common tendency in therapists to consider immediate consequences and to ignore ones occurring more distantly. For example, when a mother gives in to a child's refusal to go to school, the child ceases his distress and the mother's giving in is reinforced. However, later we may find the child watching television and enjoying his mother's company. Here the child receives further and later reinforcement (sometimes referred to as secondary gain) for his refusal behaviour. Such important consequential arrangements require attention and can only be addressed if we proceed in our exploration of the problems with questions such as, "and then what happened next?"

Details of assessment methods

Parent trainers have employed a range of assessment techniques and these have included interviews, direct observation, various questionnaires, and parent records. Here the focus of attention is on interviews and parent records.

A perusal of many texts on parent training written during the past 5–10 years shows an overwhelming preoccupation with observational methods of assessment. No doubt this resulted largely from an interest in achieving objectivity. Also, much of the parent training development occurred within research settings, where the luxury of careful and painstaking observation of interaction was feasible. Clinicians in the service sector are often unable to spare such time and must therefore rely on methods that are less time consuming. Fortunately, in recent years parent trainers have for a number of reasons shown an increased interest in interviewing.[9] Firstly, the recognition of the importance of events not readily observable, such as parental disputes and individual thinking and feeling processes, has resulted in more attention. Secondly, the realisation that success is not only about observable changes but also about changes in beliefs and attitudes (which are less immediately observable) has been influential in shaping assessment methods.

Research into interviewing methods has clearly shown that it is possible to obtain high quality factual information about family life, without necessarily hindering the important development of the therapist-client relationship (see later).[10] I would go further and state (on the basis of teaching experience), that many therapists do not realise that interviewers can gain interactional information. Practically speaking, a careful inquiry into recent behavioural episodes, sequence by sequence, can be achieved if the interviewer adopts an attitude that he would like to be able to visualise the episode in the manner of a video recording. Obviously, though such interviewing skills can never completely override the potential value of observing events, for the service clinician they can function satisfactorily as a major assessment method.

The use by parents of records of behavioural episodes serve several purposes. Further information about the problem is gained, the parents' attention is focused more specifically on the problems, and finally in consequence they can begin to observe more accurately as was mentioned earlier. Unfortunately, clinical experience indicates that parents are poor at keeping detailed records—and this is despite careful instruction and training. On visits to the clinic it is often readily apparent that their records lack detail or were completed shortly before the appointment. We can improve this by telephone checks between appointments, or by asking for audio recordings of episodes made at home, and finally the therapist can use the scanty records as a starting point for further focused interviewing as already discussed.

Issues on treatment

Careful assessment will in most instances suggest the most appropriate treatment techniques. Such assessment will include ensuring that the situations are maximally conducive to behaviour change through encouraging clear rules, ensuring that time is available to manage the problems, optimising the parents' general approach, and coaching in the use of a variety of techniques such as positive reinforcement, differential attention, time out, and point or star systems. Some discussion has already taken place with regard to things that might be changed in order to increase the probability of appropriate behaviour. The specific techniques of change are not discussed here. Rather, in this section some general and important issues relating to their application are examined.

THERAPIST SKILLS

Several research reports during the past 17 years have drawn attention to the importance of therapist skills in bringing about positive change. For instance, Alexander *et al*, in working with delinquent families, showed that a therapist's ability not only to empathise accurately, but also to direct families clearly, contributed appreciably to the likelihood of successful outcome.[11] Wahler and Dumas, in treating multiproblem families, have drawn attention to the importance of adopting a friendly, non-coercive style.[5] Finally, Patterson and colleagues (cited in Twardosz and Nordquist) have begun to examine therapist skills mainly as a consequence of inconsistent results in some of their parent training programmes.[12]

Obviously the requisite therapist skills will vary from case to case. When problems are mild and parents highly motivated, then straightforward, direct, quickly given advice may be sufficient. However, in more difficult cases the therapist will often need to create an atmosphere in which the clients feel acknowledged, supported, and encouraged to consider the resolution of their problems in a positive light. Early directing and teaching may simply drive some of these parents away. In the end, failure to give credence to the importance of therapist skills will result in resistance in therapy and possible subsequent treatment failure.

PARENTAL LEARNING OF BEHAVIOUR THERAPY TECHNIQUES

Popular books such as *Toddler Taming* contain much sound practical advice that could benefit many of the parents seen at busy outpatient clinics.[13] However, and unfortunately, many seem unable to transfer the information into action. Clearly, the distance between the written word and successful application is vast, and also such material often fails to address the distinctive nature of parent–child difficulties.

How then can parents best learn to effectively apply behavioural techniques? Several studies have shown that parents learn most effectively when techniques are role played or rehearsed and least well when the knowledge is imparted didactically.[14] The former teaching methods are time consuming, and thus in busy clinical practice we have to find some kind of reasonable balance. One possible solution is to train small groups of six to seven parents. This has been done and would appear superficially to address the time problem.[15] Additionally, working with parents in groups can in itself be facilitative, because it offers a forum in which parents can discuss and communicate their problems and solutions. Unfortunately, arranging, convening, and administering group sessions can be costly in terms of time, and this is something that is often inadequately addressed in the literature.

Another approach is to employ prepared film and video demonstrations.[12] Though this has received some attention, I would suggest that it has not been explored in this country to its full potential. Overall, we could argue that further research is required into each of these different training methods. The reality, however, is probably that the different training methods are each in their own ways effective, but that their use needs to be matched carefully to the varying needs of different clinical samples.

ANTICIPATING "ROADBLOCKS" IN TREATMENT

As has been indicated, careful assessment should hint at the optimal treatment approach and thus help reduce problems that might occur in therapy. There are, however, several commonly recurring themes within treatment that are worth addressing.

Firstly, many parents do not readily appreciate that behavioural change in themselves and their child is time consuming, and that in consequence (as is the case with learning any new skill) space and time needs to be created. For instance, in attempting to help a child develop homework skills, it is advisable as far as is possible to ensure that other household tasks occurring at the specified time take a secondary role. In all behavioural management applications it is important to discuss this with the parents with a view to encouraging maximum effort and, in consequence, reduce the negative influence of other competing events.

Secondly, standard techniques and approaches will never suit all parents. For instance, some parents might prefer to use a bedroom for "time out" and others prefer a kitchen corner. Similarly, when managing disruptive mealtime behaviour, some parents may have no difficulty in removing food until the next mealtime, but others may be unwilling to go this far. In all cases, therefore, the treatment techniques require to be presented, discussed, and then tailored to suit individual needs. Throughout such discourse one of the therapist's functions will be to ensure that what is being applied fulfills the therapeutic requirements—for example, that the positive reinforcement really is reinforcing to the child.

Thirdly, parents should be made aware that the behavioural problems may, in early treatment, increase and intensify before they improve. This is important, as some parents may read the worsening as a sign that the techniques are not working, or worse still are damaging their child. Once parents understand this point, we hope, they may read the worsening signs with encouragement and thus muster up further effort.

Fourthly, experience teaches us of some of the manipulative craft that children can exhibit during behavioural programmes. For instance, the child may adopt an "I don't care" attitude or may elicit parental guilt through statements such as "You don't love me", "You're cruel to me", etc. Viewed from a distance, the manipulative repertoires of some children can be both creative and amusing. Parents often need to be warned.

Finally, throughout treatment therapists require continually to hold the question "I wonder what might prevent successful application?" at the back of their minds. For example, how do we manage interfering adults, the presence of siblings, and the fact that parental tiredness may create difficulties in managing problems in the middle of the night?

FREQUENCY OF TREATMENT

If we are to modify successfully parent–child behaviour, then contact should be quite frequent. There is little use in initially seeing parents and children on a monthly basis. Not only do parents require frequent encouragement and support, but they also require help with early teething problems, and some of these have been referred to in the sections immediately above. At first sight this may seem to be time consuming, but much of this early work can be conducted by telephone. In fact, in many milder cases treatment may work very well with one or two clinic visits and the remainder of contact made by telephone. Once treatment has begun to succeed, then follow up at less frequent intervals is advisable for up to one year, as research findings have shown that many families require booster treatment throughout this period.[2]

EFFECT OF TREATMENT

Both clinical experience and research have shown that training parents to manage their children's behavioural problems is effective. The treatment approach would appear to work best when problems are mild, are of the acting out type, are of short duration, and where the general family background is shown to be relatively stable. Conversely, when problems are extensive, have been present for years, and occur in a context of multiple other problems, then treatments show little in the way of durable effects.[16] In cases that fall between these two extremes, the degree of success is much more difficult to assess.

The issue of calculating success rates is further compounded by

---

Summary of some important points in treatment

- Parents relate and respond better to therapists who are empathic and communicate clearly
- Treatment techniques are best learnt through observation, role play, and practice
- Changing behaviour requires time and effort
- Parents are more likely to employ techniques that suit their style and beliefs
- Behaviour often gets worse before it gets better
- Children can be very adept at frustrating change
- What will parents and children do when success occurs—in other words, what will they be able to do that they can't do now?
- During treatment brief but frequent therapist–parent contact can help prevent early treatment failures.

---

a host of variables that include the types of problems, the duration and intensity of the therapy, the quality of therapy (for example, whether therapists are experienced or newly trained), and finally what it is that actually constitutes success.

With regard to the latter point a number of issues arise. Many single case studies and reports concentrate on reductions in difficult behaviour, and neglect to mention whether or not the child shows appreciable increases in prosocial skills, generalisations of changes across environments and relationships, and changes in internal states such as might be reflected in measures of self esteem. Equally, success must be allied to how parents think, perceive, and view the situation as in the first instance they have often been responsible for the referral.

Perhaps it is unrealistic to expect much more at this time. After all, the social learning theories underpinning parent training are still largely hypothetical and our knowledge of how family events such as marital problems affect and interact with the individual child over time is still largely in its infancy. There is also a feeling that all too often the literature's use of the word success is synonymous with cure. Kendall quite rightly asserts that the notion that people can be "fixed" is unreasonable and unhelpful.[17] For instance, if our successfully treated school refuser returns with further problems three years later, this is not necessarily indicative of past failure, but rather indicates that more therapy is required. The conclusion we can draw is that if we can be helpful at one moment in time then our function becomes more realistic, credible, and healthy.

Concluding remarks

This brief examination of parent training in behavioural child management has focused on only some aspects considered important by a practising clinician. Many topics have not even been considered. These, among others, include observational methodology, common treatment techniques such as time out and differential attention, contingency contracting procedures, coping and problem solving strategies, and a range of adjunctive treatment procedures designed to improve and enhance outcome. For further information the reader is referred to a number of useful source books listed in the appendix.

Most developments in parent training have taken place in research settings, and there is an urgent need to conduct efficacy studies in the routine clinical sector to establish how the technology will stand up when time is short and caseloads are large. It is to be hoped that the new emphasis on medical and clinical audit will serve as well in this direction over the next decade and beyond

1 Ollendick TH. Child and adolescent behaviour therapy. In: Garfield JL, Bergin AE, eds. *Handbook of psychotherapy and behaviour change*. New York: Wiley, 1986:525–64.

2 Patterson GR, Reid JB, Jones RR, Couger RE. *A social learning approach to family interventions: families with aggressive children*. Eugene, Oregon: Castalia, 1975.

3 Jenkins JM, Smith MA. Marital disharmony and children's behaviour problems: aspects of a poor marriage that affect children adversely. *J Child Psychol Psychiatry* 1991;32:793–810.

4 Wallerstein J, Corbin SB, Lewis JM. Children of divorce: a ten-year study. In: Hetherington EM, Arastch J, eds. *Impact of divorce, single parenting and stepparenting on children*. Hillsdale, New Jersey: Erlbaum, 1989:202–14.

5 Wahler RG, Dumas JE. Changing the observational coding styles of insular and noninsular mothers: a step towards maintenance of parent training effects. In: Dangel RF, Polster RA, eds. *Parent training: foundations of research and practice*. New York: Guilford, 1984:379–416.

6 Wolfe DA. Child abuse. In: Hersen M, Hasselt VB, eds. *Behavior therapy with children and adolescents*. New York: Wiley, 1987:385–415.

7 Wolfe DA. *Child abuse*. London: Sage, 1987.

8 Webster-Stratton C, Hammond M. Maternal depression and its relationship to life stress, perceptions and child behavior problems, parenting behaviors, and child conduct problems. *J Abnorm Child Psychol* 1988;16:299–315.

9 Mash EJ, Terdal LG. Behavioral assessment of child and family disturbance. In: Mash EJ, Terdal LG, eds. *Behaviour assessment of childhood disorders*. New York: Guilford, 1988:3–65.

10 Cox A, Rutter M. Diagnostic appraisal and interviewing. In: Rutter M, Hersov L, eds. *Child and adolescent psychiatry: modern approaches*. Oxford: Blackwell, 1985:233–48.

11 Alexander JF, Barton C, Schiavo RS, Parsons BV. Systems behavioral intervention with families of delinquents: therapist characteristics, family behavior and outcome. *J Consult Clin Psychol* 1976;44:656–64.

12 Twardosz S, Nordquist VM. Parent training. In: Hersen M, Van Hasselt VB, eds. *Behavior therapy with children and adolescents*. New York: John Wiley, 1987.

13 Green C. *Toddler taming*. London: Doubleday, 1990.

14 O'Dell SL, O'Quin JA, Alford BA, O'Briant AL, Bradlyn AS, Giebenhain JC. Predicting the acquisition of parenting skills via four training methods. *Behavior Therapy* 1982;**13**:194–208.

15 O'Dell SL. Progress in parent training. In: Hersen N, Eisler RM, Miller PM, eds. *Progress behavior modification*. New York: Academic Press, 1985:57–108.

16 Wahler RG, Graves MG. Setting events in social networks: ally or enemy in child behavior therapy. *Behavior Therapy* 1983:19–36.

17 Kendall PC. The generalization and maintenance of behavior change: comments, considerations, and the "no-cure" criticism. *Behavior Therapy* 1989:357–64.

Appendix

The child behaviour therapy books listed are ones that I have found most useful. This list is by no means exhaustive, but should provide readers with a fairly broad coverage of the field of child behaviour therapy.

CHILD BEHAVIOUR ASSESSMENT

The one text listed here, which is now in its second edition, is authoritative and has become a standard bench book. In addition to chapters on conduct, emotional, and developmental problems, there are also chapters on brain injury, chronic pain, obesity, anorexia nervosa, enuresis, encopresis, child abuse, and other subjects. The breadth of coverage has hitherto been unusual in behaviourally oriented textbooks.

Mash EJ, Terdal LG, eds. *Behavioral assessment of childhood disorders*. New York: Guilford, 1988.

THERAPIST HANDBOOKS

The two books here provide therapists with detailed guidelines for conducting child behaviour therapy assessment, treatment planning, treatment implementation, and outcome evaluation. Both texts are practical and contain a wealth of clinical experience.

Herbert M. *Behavioural treatment of problem children*. London: Academic Press, 1981.
Herbert M. *Working with children and their families*. London: Routledge, 1988.

CHILD BEHAVIOUR THERAPY HANDBOOKS

The two books listed deal with a wide range of different childhood disorders and problems. I prefer the second text, mainly because of its masterly coverage of vast areas of behaviour therapy literature. Unfortunately this text is now rapidly becoming rather dated.

Hersen M, Van Hasselt VB, eds. *Behavior therapy with children and adolescents.* New York: Wiley, 1987.

Ross AO. *Child behavior therapy: principles, procedures and empirical basis.* New York: Wiley, 1981.

CHILD BEHAVIOURAL MANAGEMENT MANUALS

The three books listed provide basic information on the management of a range of child behavioural problems. Generally they are fairly straightforward and not too laden with technical jargon. I prefer the first book as it not only contains much practical management advice but it also addresses many of the practical problems encountered in counselling parents.

Barkely RA. *Defiant children.* New York: Guilford, 1990.

Green C. *Toddler taming.* London: Doubleday, 1990.

Patterson GR. *Families.* Champaign, Illinois: Research Press, 1977.

5. Family therapy: change the family, change the child?

Christopher Dare

Definition

The psychological health and the normal course of development of a child are closely determined by the nature of the security, predictability, and appropriateness of the immediate social environment. For most children, in Western postindustrial culture, this environment centres on the nuclear family. Over the past four decades there has evolved a psychotherapeutic intervention that takes family life as its subject matter. This is now known, simply, as family therapy.* In its earlier stages it was designated whole family therapy or family group therapy.

Application and effects of family therapy

Family therapy has become a widespread clinical practice within child and adolescent psychiatry. The research basis for this extensive application is slim, as is the case for most psychotherapeutic methods. There are also problems in the interpretation of the research: "In sum, the search for an assessment of family therapy effectiveness has been frustrated by a research base that past reviewers have found difficult to synthesize".[1] Hence, the justification for the use of family therapy in child psychiatric settings is largely based on "clinical experience"†: it appears sensible to

* Throughout this chapter the word family refers to the household of a family of creation. That is to say, it consists of a parent or parents with children for whom the adults are responsible for the foreseeable future. Other members of the household related or unrelated by blood may be included in a therapy session.
† Gurman and Kniskern point out that the efficacy of family therapy is best established in the form of marital therapy for marital problems.[2] Clearly, many children are seriously troubled by parental discord and marital therapy is not, therefore, irrelevant to child health professionals. However, any discussion of marital therapy is beyond the range of this chapter.

52

approach problems of behaviour and effective disturbance through the family context.

None the less, in reviewing evidence for the efficacy of family therapy, Gurman and Kniskern report that the usefulness of family therapy is established for behavioural and emotional disturbance in childhood and adolescence.[2] Likewise, in the review of Hazelrigg et al there is a conclusion, from a meta-analytic study of a number of control trials of family therapy, that it can be shown to be more effective than no treatment or control treatments.[1] Most of the effective treatments reported by these authors, where the presenting problem is described, concern children with behaviour problems. Patterson has reported extensively on the effectiveness of his form of family intervention, based on social learning theory in behavioural disorder in primary school aged children (see previous chapter).[3] Alexander and Barton showed the effectiveness of another form of family therapy (using an admixture of systems and behavioural theory) in the management of behaviourally disturbed children.[4] Lask and Matthews have shown the usefulness of family therapy as an adjunct to physical treatments in asthma.[5] (The therapy here was "structural" in form.) Ro-Trock et al have shown that family therapy added to the milieu treatments in an adolescent unit improves the benefits of the inpatient regimen.[6] In our own studies at the Institute of Psychiatry we have shown that family therapy is superior to a supportive individual therapy in the management of anorexia in adolescence.[7][8] Our as yet unpublished findings show that the benefits of family therapy, compared with the control treatment, persists at five year follow up. Our family therapy can be designated as including psychoanalytic as well as structural and strategic elements.[9]

In addition to family therapy being used in the management of a child's presenting problems, it has also been used to alleviate family distress and to optimise family functioning in chronic physical illness.[10] In principle, family therapy is to be considered as part of the treatment plan in a wide range of chronic and distressing childhood illness.

In the course of this introduction, defining labels have been attached to reported outcome studies. This is necessary as there are many forms of family therapy. Although there have been very few studies of the specific strengths and applications of the different schools of family therapy, it is necessary to describe them in order to understand the diversity of techniques used within the therapy. Examination of the origins of family therapy and the context in which it developed provides a way of defining the different theoretical origins and styles of current practice.

Origins of family therapy

Family therapy grew from dissatisfaction with the psychotherapeutic techniques that were available in the 1950s.[11] In the early 1950s therapeutic techniques of psychoanalytic psychotherapy and psychodynamic casework were, essentially, the only well established treatment methods in child psychiatry departments and in child guidance clinics. These techniques came to be applied to the child and to the two parents, so that in a well staffed clinic three professionals were involved in the treatment of one case. Such treatments, usually long term, if carried out conscientiously led to the discovery that psychological difficulties existed for other children in the family than the first one to be presented. A fourth or even a fifth therapist might be recruited to the management of what had been, in the first instance, one case. Three problems arose: firstly, this technical development of multiple therapists was hopelessly uneconomic. Secondly, there were difficulties in coordinating the different therapies. Thirdly, the unavailability of most child mental health problems to such intensive therapy was obvious as family resistance to long term psychotherapy became apparent.[12]

Family therapy began to be applied pragmatically to children's problems in the decade after the second world war.[13-15] The concepts and techniques largely resembled a psychodynamic group therapy with some psychodrama (in the therapies of Ackerman).

However, another context, derived from the second world war, had a unique and crucial influence. The Veterans Administration (VA) was responsible for the health care of the former conscripts into the US armed forces. Given the age group and numbers of men recruited into the forces, and the stresses that they endured, it was not surprising that, in the postwar period, the VA found itself looking after a large number of young men with psychotic illnesses, which were at that time largely untreatable. Modern psychopharmacological agents were not available and a few heroic experiments in the psychotherapy of these patients were yielding poor results.

The National Institute of Mental Health (NIMH) and the VA at Palo Alto set up research programmes investigating the families of young adult schizophrenic patients. The NIMH research[16] and the VA group both had long term effects not upon the development of a family therapy effective in the management of schizophrenia, but on the conceptual framework and practices of the family therapy in child mental health settings.[17][18] Both groups observed processes within the family as a whole.

The NIMH used psychological tests on all family members (the thematic apperception test, a projective test akin to the Rorschach ink blots) and identified discrepancies between verbal meaning and the affective implications of communication in families such as "pseudomutuality" and "pseudohostility". Pseudomutuality refers to a communication in which an overt warmth belies an underlying antagonism, whereas pseudohostility implies a closeness overlaid with an apparent hostility.

The Palo Alto VA group looked at the family as it sat talking together with a member of the research team. The VA group was remarkable in that it drew upon unusual talents: Jay Haley, a communications expert; Geoffrey Bateson, a cultural anthropologist; Virginia Satir, a social case worker; and Don Jackson, a psychoanalyst, a follower of the American founder of 'interpersonal' psychoanalysis Harry Stacks Sullivan. All of these made distinctive contributions that have shaped modern family therapy. For example, Haley as a communications expert was specifically interested in the patterns of verbal and non-verbal communication. Bateson from previous anthropological field studies had experience of the discrepancy between overt and covert communication and its effects upon social behaviour.[19] Jackson was skilled in construing the nature of the psychological effects of one family on each other and in mobilising psychotherapeutic interventions that addressed these effects. Satir drew on knowledge of family and group processes observed in social work practice. The well known but inaccurately understood "double bind" form of communication summarised some of the group's views.[20] In the "double bind" situation a pronounced discrepancy between overt verbal communication and the covert emotional context is complicated by the imposition of an additional rule that prohibits reference to the discrepancy.

Family systems theory and family therapy

The distinctive contribution of the Palo Alto research group derived from the introduction of systems theory[21] and ecology[22]

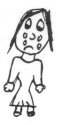

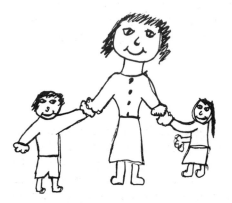

What it feels like to be left out: 11 year old. Family therapy can improve the general satisfaction of family members with their life together

into an understanding of families. The family members' mutual dependence and influence on each other was seen to create a system that had properties in its own right which were not necessarily predictable from the qualities of the individuals ("the whole is greater than the sum of the individual parts"). This concept, that the family could be defined as a totality, had a momentous effect on the development of family therapy, far beyond the potential usefulness of family therapy in the management of schizophrenia in young adults. It has become incorporated as a "family systems theory" approach.

The Palo Alto group dispersed (after the early death of Jackson) but came to influence family therapy, turning it from a marginal activity of a small group of child mental health workers to a major movement in contemporary thinking about families and children.

The family therapy movement has become synonymous with the concepts of family systems theory. As such it has had a large impact on child and adolescent psychiatric practice and is beginning to influence studies of child development[23][24] and the scientific study of interpersonal relations.[25]

Family therapy techniques and practice

Despite the percolation of family systems thinking into empirical studies, family therapy remains, like much of psychotherapy, a practice driven by clinical observation and experience rather than by scientific studies. Despite the fact that systematic reports of treatment trials[7] and of family systems investigations[26] are occurring, the descriptions of most family therapy practice rely upon accounts derived from clinical know how. Contemporary family therapy can be described under the headings of "schools" of practice.

Strategic family therapy

The roots of much modern psychotherapy lie in psychoanalysis with its tradition of listening, non-directiveness, and a belief in the therapeutic potency of insight promoting interpretation. The growth of other psychological treatments based on empirical psychology, especially learning theory, challenged these tenets of psychoanalysis. However, even before behaviour therapy had become well known, Haley as a family therapist (1963) had proposed that psychotherapy could be directive and goal orientated and he coined the phrase "strategic" therapy.[11] What he meant by this was that the therapist had a responsibility to identify the end point of treatment, which should then be sought by whatever means. The viewpoint tends to be associated with a mistrust of theory based treatment goals and takes the problem, as presented by the patient or the family consensus, as the principle guide to the direction of treatment. Hence if the family nominate the child's faecal soiling as the problem then the therapist helps the family devise strategies to eliminate the soiling. The problem as stated *is* the problem, not a putative underlying psychopathology of the individual or of the family. This particular approach to therapy has been definitively described by Haley[27] and it characterises most therapies, especially those that are short term. It is especially relevant to work with young children and with acute problems.

Almost any technique that can produce change can be called upon in the pursuit of a potent strategy to augment the power of the family over the problem. For example behavioural therapy techniques (especially the keeping of a diary of the unwanted and

wanted behaviours), quasihypnotic suggestion, challenging interpretations and so on, may all be used. Some of the most striking
methods are labelled as paradoxical interventions. The therapist
raises the family's anxiety by suggesting that the symptom may
have to get worse, remain indefinitely, or be deliberately enacted.
Commonly, a persuasive rationale for the suggestion may be given.
Such techniques may have an effect by increasing the family's
determination to counteract the problem or its effects. Likewise,
the child with the symptom may be helped to feel more in control
of the problem when instructed to perform the symptomatic
behaviour deliberately. For example, an enuretic child may be
advised to wet the bed deliberately ("You choose a time when the
flood can be best dealt with"). Or the whole family might be
encouraged to take on a symptom: a tic, nervous cough, or
whatever. The use of strategic techniques, like all family therapy,
is embedded within an approach to the family that is positive,
supportive, and non-critical. The therapist tries to put the family
into a frame of mind that will enable them to take charge of the
symptom, if not immediately, in the longer term.

Structural family therapy

The great achievement of the Palo Alto group had been to
produce a language whereby the space *between* the family members
was attended to as much as to processes *within* the individuals
themselves. That is to say the family was described as a whole, as
an organisation with identifiable rules and structure.

A family can be defined as existing to provide psychological
support, companionship, and fulfilment to the adults (if there is
more than one parent in the family) and to nurture children from
infancy to young adulthood. To achieve these there must be
systems of communication, of control, of nurturance, and of affect
management. There have to be rules governing the balance of
selfish and altruistic behaviour as well as establishing the demands
of intimacy and separateness. Family members have different roles
usually determined, in part, by age, gender, state of physical and
psychological health, and by family traditions. A family has
implicitly a definition of who is inside and who outside the family
and of maintaining the distinction between the two areas. All of
these aspects are especially important in inducing children into
membership of the family and contribute appreciably to the
personality of the growing child. As these aspects are examined

and specified for different families the structure of a particular family is being described.

All family therapy, by definition, attempts to change the structure of the family, but a particular group of family therapists has taken such change as its specific aim. This school centres around the teaching of Salvador Minuchin especially that emanating from the Philadelphia child guidance clinic.[28][29] Minuchin was most interested in the hierarchical structure of families, in the coalitions between family members, in the clarity or otherwise of its rules and controls, and in the clarity or otherwise of the boundaries between individual family members. In the form of family therapy associated with Minuchin, the therapist construes a symptom as being an expression of a disorder of family organisation. Society and individual needs are taken to be best met by families with an optimal organisation. If that organisation does not pertain, dysfunction in the family can be said to occur and disturbance ensues in the individual. The therapy, in seeking to identify and reverse family dysfunction, facilitates the relief of the individual bearing the symptom.

Stated in this simplified way there are obvious dangers to structural family therapy in seeking to define socially determined organisations as "normal" and the reverse as "abnormal". The main thrust of much structural family therapy is to clarify and enhance parental authority over the children, to strengthen the marital couple in their rule setting, and to make the children more separate from and subject to the parents.

The structural therapist functions by adding professional authority to that of the parents. Instructions and directions are given to the parents as to how they should conduct family life with more clarity of organisation. Tasks are prescribed that, in their completion between sessions, will continue to augment the precision of family rules and to give the family practice in their maintenance. Such activities are manifestly beneficial, if successful, in chaotic and under-organised families.[30] Such structurally based interventions are also sensible in families where there is an apparent ideology of democracy that leaves children confused as to what are the differences between children and adults and what are the rules expected of them inside and outside the family. Most families lie between the extremes of chaos and ill placed democracy but none the less the techniques of structural therapy are widely applicable. A "family diagnosis" will always attend to enduring structural qualities.

Behavioural family therapy

Many family therapists, as has been made clear in the descriptions so far, are directed towards explicit behaviours and, as such, have implicitly accepted the underlying principles of behaviour therapy. Some family therapists have made a wholehearted adaptation of behavioural practices to whole family intervention.[3 31] Such an approach will clearly be akin to aspects of the strategic, problem solving approach in that the unwanted behaviour will be accepted as the problem. A very detailed behavioural analysis will be made, the pattern of antecedent and subsequent events will be carefully investigated, and the frequency and timing of the problem behaviours identified by, for example, a diary. The symptom is attacked, directly, by alteration of the behavioural contingencies; the family is taught to ignore unwanted behaviour and to reward wanted alternatives systematically and enthusiastically.

Such an approach can be highly effective with troublesome misbehaviour, especially in young children. However, the effectiveness of such an approach extends beyond simple behavioural management. Many children presenting with problems ranging as widely as conduct disorder, depression, somatic disorders, or phobias may have poor self esteem. This can be continually reinforced both by the manifestations of the child's disturbance but also by the parents' sense of failure and helplessness consequent on their child's difficulties. It is easy for families to get into a cycle of blame and recrimination, and the implementation of a simple behavioural programme as described can alter the family atmosphere. The parents and other children are directed to be positive and approving of what is acceptable while ignoring the negative and unacceptable.

Falloon has used behavioural notions of social skills and problem solving to help families with a schizophrenic member.[31] Epstein and Bishop have elaborated a programme, the McMaster's model, that likewise uses a great deal of direct behavioural instruction to change identified areas of apparent family dysfunction as well as individual misbehaviour.[32]

Transgenerational family therapy

So far the emphasis has been on techniques that are widely used in family therapy and that are distinct from the mainstream of psychodynamic psychotherapy that dominates individual therapy. It can be argued that these differences are more apparent than real,[9] [33] [34] but in the description of family therapy given so far the emphasis has been on the family as an organisation that is defined by its transactional qualities: by those qualities that are directly observable or construable from the current pattern of interaction between family members.

However, a family also has a history. The parent (or parents) has experienced family life during childhood and will draw on those experiences in forming a new family. A child's experiences of nurturance and the formation of attachments will come into play, when the child is now adult, in the pattern of bonding and loving in the new family.[35] Bowen,[36] Framo,[37] and Byng-Hall[38] have described a variety of techniques whereby the family therapist calls on the history of the family to gain therapeutic power.

The tool of the transgenerational family therapist is the construction and examination of a family tree (also known as a geneogram). In this process each family member is asked to cooperate in the actual drawing of a family tree. Often it is most advantageous to ask the least involved, most disengaged family member to tell of the present family and its forebears. Likewise, it may be sensible to ask designated patients, the "naughty" children, about the family story so that they can show their affiliation by their knowledge and interest in that story. As the family members tell the therapist about who makes up the family and its genealogy, questions about the perceived personality and relationships of that individual can be discussed.

Different viewpoints illustrate generational and gender perspectives and allow the therapist to endorse the sense of family membership, of loyalty, and of the normality of difference. The technique of drawing up a family tree is akin to psychodynamic work because it allows for the interpretation of rules, of patterns, of unconscious and conscious identifications, and so on. At the same time, the manner in which the therapist addresses the family can support and strengthen the family's hierarchical strength and intergenerational boundaries and so "structural" work can be done.

Milan systems family therapy

Most of the techniques described so far have required the therapist to be rather active, to give strong direction to the therapy, and to invite the family to change by doing things differently. Such a style of therapy is most obviously appropriate for short term treatments, for those brought about by urgent problems, and for those cases in which the presenting problem is the management of misbehaviour in children.

There are other situations, in which the therapy must be more reflective, exploratory, and more ambiguous in its ostensible aims. There are also therapists whose personal style tends more in these directions. Such a style resembles more the practice of psycho-analytic psychotherapy and it is not surprising that a form of family therapy embodying some of these qualities has evolved. What is less predictable is that this school has been extremely influential throughout the field of family therapy.

This school was initiated by the Italian psychiatrist/psychother-apist, Mara Selvini-Palazzoli. Because she worked and taught in Milan and because early in her move from individual to family therapy she was strongly influenced by Bateson, her school has become known as that of Milan systems therapy. Selvini-Palazzoli has outlined the development of her theory[39] and her co-workers and followers have written extensively on the methods of what has now become a worldwide school.

The Milan systems therapist does not seek to produce change by deliberately directing or restructuring the family. Instead the therapist tries to evolve an analysis of the family's history and relationship patterns by asking a series of questions that invite the family to reflect on their own and each other's experiences of their lives together. The aim is to expose the assumptions that underlie the attitudes and behaviour patterns of the family. This exposure, when successfully facilitated, leads the family itself to attempt new ways of relating to and treating each other without direct sugges-tions coming from the therapist. In passing, it can be noted that many of the interpretations that Milan systems therapists use to understand families are *transgenerational*, emphasising, for ex-ample, the rigid loyalty that families may show in adhering to particular patterns that determine the family organisation.

Common themes in family therapy practice

In the development of family therapy the designation of dis-tinctive schools has been important in helping different ideas to be pursued rigorously and extensively, but it has also led to counter-productive notions of orthodoxies and to competitiveness. Al-though the distinctive schools persist, the average practitioner will use a mixture of ideas and techniques derived from a variety of schools. Nichols, among others, has propounded the view that the

---

Treatment strategies in family therapy

- Strategic: targets symptom change
- Structural: aims to change or restructure the family (in relation to parental authority, rule setting, and individuation)
- Behavioural: uses behavioural techniques
- Transgenerational: calls on the history of the family to gain therapeutic power (psychodynamic understanding and use of "family trees"; it allows for the interpretation of rules, patterns, and identifications within the family; it supports family hierarchy and intergenerational boundaries)
- Milan systems therapy: aims to explore the assumptions underlying attitudes and behavioural patterns in the family.

---

different schools of family therapy share more than their adherents sometimes acknowledge.[40] The mixture that forms a particular therapist's style will depend on the training, reading, and personal qualities of the therapist.

There are regular themes in these eclectic therapies. In principle, all family therapies aspire to change family structures, but respect hierarchical organisations and the differing needs of children and adults. All family therapies accept that the family will need to be engaged by a discussion of what they perceive to be the problem. Most family therapists accept that patterns of family functioning are transmitted from one generation to another, resulting in what can be called a *family culture*. All family therapists will observe ethnocultural sensibilities.

Concept of the family life cycle

One particular concept shared by most family therapists is that a family is an evolving, growing structure going through distinctive stages with transitions denoting the move from one phase to another. This is the basis for the concept of the *family life cycle*, a major theme in all family therapy and relevant to any practitioner wishing to consider the family of a child.[33 41]

The main implication of the concept is that at different phases in the evolution of a particular family there are likely to be characteristic tasks and preoccupations. For example, the family can be said to begin when a couple choose, or have forced upon them, the necessity to accommodate a child. The couple is a two person organisation, principally involved in the creation of a mutually supportive and enhancing personal relationship. The arrival of a baby demands a family unit organised around the need to maintain the biological integrity and healthy development of an infant. The couple's need as a pair takes second place.

The pace of family adaptation becomes dominated by the changing needs for protection and nurturance of the infant growing from babyhood to schoolchildhood. At the point of entrance to whole time education there begins a period when, although child care remains a dominant activity, the parents' attention to their own interests and ambitions can increase. The school age child changes as he or she matures, contributing a share to the changing needs of the family, and this process is accelerated as adolescence is reached and the potential for adulthood is signalled in the child. This requires further family adaptation and offers the possibility of more freedom for the parents. However, in childhood, the pace of change in the family tends to be dominated by the rate of development of children.

The life cycle does not come to a halt in adulthood. The changes of midlife and of old age impinge on families, especially for young families, in the lives of the grandparents. The greater the number of people in the family going through major life cycle transitions, the greater the demand for change that is imposed on the family as a whole. These demands for change are potentially stressful and family therapy can be seen as centering around the process of acquisition of skills to overcome these stresses.

Contraindications and side effects

Little work as been done that can give an informed account of contraindications to family therapy. In a published study I and colleagues have shown that high levels of family criticism predict poor outcome of family therapy in adolescents with restricting eating disorder.[47] This effect can possibly be counteracted by specific interventions to reduce such criticism. In general, family therapy is much more difficult in families where there is great unhappiness and dissatisfaction with family life, but this is not an automatic contraindication to the treatment. There is certainly good evidence that couple therapy can improve the quality of the relationship, and family therapy could possibly improve the general satisfaction of family members with their life together. These considerations are relevant to the discussion of the side effects of family therapy. Families regularly complain that family therapy disturbs them. Conflicts that have been hidden might become overt. It is very common for the parents of a disturbed child to believe that their marital disagreements are a cause of the disturbance. Defensively, a couple may come to believe that the family therapy has caused the marital disagreement that, in fact, antedates attendance for treatment. These occurrences make it difficult for clinicians to identify genuine, negative side effects of family therapy. This is an area where systematic study is needed.

Conclusion

All clinicians working with children will know the importance of the family's influence in determining the care of children and the management of their psychosocial life. Common sense, both social and clinical, will enable most problems to be handled by most of us. However, from time to time, common sense is of no use and then uncommon solutions are necessary. That is often the case where there are psychological problems in childhood whether arising *ab initio* or deriving from other difficulties such as chronic illness. Family therapy has some of the qualities of uncommon sense: convening a whole family meeting to discover solutions to problems does not come naturally to professionals or to patients. However, many of the techniques of family therapy are clinically cogent and are powerful influences on family behaviour. These powers can be harnessed for the good of children in our professional care.

The author's research described in this chapter has been generously supported by the Medical Research Council of Great Britain.

1 Hazelrigg MD, Cooper HM, Bourdin CM. Evaluating the effectiveness of family therapy: an integrative review and analysis. *Psychol Bull* 1987;**101**:428–42.
2 Gurman AS, Kniskern DP. Family therapy outcome research: knowns and unknowns. In: Gurman AS, Kniskern DP, eds. *Handbook of family therapy*. New York: Brunner/Mazel, 1981:742–51.
3 Patterson GR. Behavioral intervention procedures in the classroom and the home. In: Bergin AE, Garfield SL, eds. *Handbook of psychotherapy and behavior change*. New York: Wiley, 1979.
4 Alexander J, Barton C. Behavioral systems therapy with delinquent families. In: Olson DH, ed. *Treating relationships*. Lake Mills, Indiana: Graphic, 1976:656–64.
5 Lask B, Matthews D. Childhood asthma: a controlled trial of family therapy. *Arch Dis Child* 1979;**54**:116–9.
6 Ro-Trock C, Wellisch D, Schroder J. A family therapy outcome in an in-patient setting. *Am J Orthopsychiatry* 1977;**47**:514–22.
7 Russell GFM, Szmukler G, Dare C, Eisler I. An evaluation of family therapy in anorexia nervosa and bulimia nervosa. *Arch Gen Psychiatry* 1987;**44**:1047–56.

8 Dare C, Eisler I, Russell GFM, Szmukler G. The clinical and theoretical impact of a controlled trial of family therapy in anorexia nervosa. *Journal of Marital and Family Therapy* 1900;**16**:39–57.

9 Dare C. Psychoanalytic family therapy. In: Street E, Dryden W, eds. *Family therapy in Britain*. Milton Keynes: Open University Press, 1988:23–50.

10 Kazak AE, Nachmann GS. Famil research on childhood chronic illness: paediatric oncology as an example. *Journal of Family Psychology* 1991;**4**:462–83.

11 Haley J. *Strategies of psychotherapy*. New York: Grune and Stratton, 1963.

12 Minuchin S. Psychoanalytic therapies and the low socio–economic population. In: Marmor J, ed. *Modern psychoanalysis*. New York: Basic Books, 1970:532–50.

13 Bowlby J. The study and reduction of group tension in the family. *Human Relations* 1949;**2**:123–8.

14 Bell JE. Recent advances in family group therapy. *J Child Psychol Psychiatry* 1962;**3**:1–15.

15 Ackerman NW. *The psychodynamics of family life*. New York: Basic Books, 1958.

16 Wynne LC, Singer MT. Thought disorder and family relations of schizophrenics. I: a research strategy. *Arch Gen Psychiatry* 1963;**9**:191–8.

17 Jackson DD, ed. *Communication, family, and marriage*. Palo Alto: Science and Behavior Books, 1968.

18 Jackson DD, ed. *Therapy, communication, and change*. Palo Alto: Science and Behavior Books, 1969.

19 Bateson G. *Steps to an ecology of mind*. London: Paladin, 1973.

20 Bateson G, Jackson DD, Haley J, Weakland JH. A note on the double bind. *Fam Process* 1963;**2**:154–61.

21 Von Bertalanffy I. The theory of open systems in physics and biology. In: Emery FE, ed. *Systems thinking*. Harmondworth: Penguin, 1950:23–7.

22 Waddington CH. *Tools for thought*. London: Jonathan Cape, 1977.

23 Sander L. Investigations of the infant and its care-giving environment as a biological system. In: Greenspan SI, Pollock GH, eds. *The course of life*. Vol 1. Washington DC: National Institutes of Mental Health, 1980:177–201.

24 Tyson P, Tyson RL. *Psychoanalytic theories of development*. New Haven: Yale University Press, 1991.

25 Hinde RA, Stevenson-Hinde J, eds. *Relationships within families: mutual influences*. Oxford: Clarendon Press, 1988.

26 Eisler I, Szmukler G, Dare C. Systematic observation and clinical insight: are they compatible? An experiment in recognizing family interaction. *Psychol Med* 1985;**15**:701–37.

27 Haley J. *Problem-solving therapy*. San Francisco: Jossey-Bass, 1976.

28 Minuchin S. *Families and family therapy*. Cambridge, Massachusetts: Harvard University Press, 1974.

29 Minuchin S, Fishman C. *Family therapy techniques*. Cambridge, Massachusetts: Harvard University Press, 1981.

30 Umbarger CC. *Structural family therapy*. New York: Grune and Stratton, 1983.

31 Falloon IM. *Handbook of behavioural family therapy*. London: Unwin Hyman, 1988.

32 Epstein NB, Bishop DS. Problem centred systems therapy of the family. In: Gurman AS, Kniskern DP, eds. *Handbook of Family Therapy*. New York: Brunner/Mazel, 1981.

33 Dare C. Psychoanalysis and systems in family therapy. *Journal of Family Therapy* 1979;**1**:137–56.

34 Dare C. Psychoanalysis and family therapy. In: Walrond Skinner S, ed. *Developments in family therapy*. London: Routledge and Kegan Paul, 1981:281–97.

35 Doane JA, Hill WL jnr, Diamond D. A developmental view of therapeutic bonding in the family: the treatment of the disconnected family. *Fam Process* 1991;**30**:155–75.
36 Bowen M. *Family therapy in clinical practice.* New York: Jason Aronson, 1978.
37 Framo JL. *Explorations in marital and family therapy.* New York: Springer, 1982.
38 Byng-Hall J. Family legends: their significance for the family therapist. In: Bentovim A, Gorell Barnes G, Cooklin A. eds. *Family therapy: complementary framework of theory and practice.* London: Academic Press, 1982:213–28.
39 Selvini-Palazzoli M. *Self starvation: from the intraphysic to the transpersonal approach.* London: Chaucer, 1974.
40 Nichols N. *Family therapy: concepts and methods.* New York: Gardner, 1984.
41 Carter EA, McGoldrick M, eds. *The family life cycle: a framework for family therapy.* New York: Gardner Press, 1980.
42 Le Grange D, Eisler I, Dare C, Hodes M. Family criticism and self-starvation: a study of expressed emotion. *Journal of Family and Marital Therapy* 1992;**14**:177–92.

6. Group psychotherapy for children and adolescents

S Reid, I Kolvin

Definition

By definition, group psychotherapy involves a therapist or cotherapists treating several children in groups. There are two main theoretical approaches—psychodynamic and behavioral or cognitive. The latter distinction is not necessarily a clear cut one, and a rather simplistic view would be that whereas "behavioural" psychotherapy in children seeks directly to alter surface behaviour, "psychodynamic" psychotherapy is more geared to helping children towards a deeper understanding of their own behaviour. In this chapter we address ourselves to the psychodynamic approach.

The original version of group psychotherapy was "activity" group therapy[1] which, although based on psychodynamic principles, tended not to use techniques of interpretation but focused on activity, appreciating that some young children could reveal themselves better in play and activity than in discussion. Group "play" therapy developed by Axline[2] using Rogers' non-directive principles[3] has been used widely in community settings.[4] In this version, expression of feelings are facilitated in the younger children; the therapist is reflective but not directive, and hence the play is not directed beyond the limits necessary to allow the therapy to continue within the clinic or other setting. For example, the children must stay in the room and are expected not to destroy the fabric of the room or to hurt each other physically. One of the main centres for the development of group therapy with children in the United Kingdom is the Tavistock Clinic; their model emerged out of psychodynamic theory, following the work of Klein[5-8] and Bion[9 10] and is described elsewhere.[11 12]

However, even within each approach there may be variations and thus the approach used is likely to be determined by the training of the therapist and the nature of the problems addressed. Therapy as described in this paper is based on an understanding of group dynamics, with the main impact being in the context of the "here and now" situation, with a focus on the personality and behaviour of each child, the relationship between peers, and the nature of each child's relationship with the therapist, rather than an exploration of early life events. The therapist seeks to create an atmosphere that allows each child to feel accepted and respected by the therapist for the person she or he is. A setting is provided that can be experienced by the group as safe and reliable and which enables the exploration of combinations of relationships, dysfunctional communication, and unconscious processes. Group psychotherapy recognises that all children have a range of strengths as well as weaknesses, and an appreciation of this by children has a potential for therapeutic impact on other group members.

The therapeutic aim is to enable four or five *younger* children, or six to nine *older* children or adolescents, to become a group. With younger children the approach in essence may be that of psychodynamically orientated group therapy with a focus on following play principles outlined by several group therapists[13-16] and with older children and adolescents with the focus on verbal interactions.[3] In becoming a group, the individuals need to recognise and value the uniqueness and sovereignty of each of the other members, and to come to understand those others as also representing aspects of themselves.[15] The group provides an opportunity to explore and capitalise on interactions between peers, the children, and the therapist(s), as well as both present and past interpersonal experiences and family relationships. In this model the therapist may set limits, may interpret interactions, and seeks to promote an understanding of social skills and peer relationships.

The nature of the group

It has often been asserted that a group is more than a mere collection of individuals but, rather, that the members have a common task and come to identify with the group and its aims and are thus interdependent. In addition, Freud argued that the fundamental component of the group was a leader.[17] However, social psychologists offer other definitions of groups, such as "a social unit consisting of a number of individuals who stand in role

69

and status relationships to one another, stabilised in some degree at the time, and who possess a set of values or norms of their own regulating their behaviour, at least in matters of consequence to the group".[18] The latter definition implies that some individuals are inside, whereas others are outside the group; this gives rise to a sense of group cohesiveness for those within the group. However, such cohesiveness may be in danger of potential disruption by "disturbing motives" of individual members, such as a wish to have the therapist to oneself or angry feelings about other group members. Such disturbing motives need to be explored within the group to enable members to find a constructive or helpful solution. Other theorists argue that the behaviour of clients in therapy groups is governed by a balance of emotional forces.[19]

Some ways in which groups may be therapeutic

It is important to try to understand the ways in which groups may be therapeutic, especially in relation to children, and Yalom makes a major contribution to this.[20] He identifies several themes, and we address those particularly relevant to children: (a) the instillation of a sense of hope, (b) children have a considerable need to "belong", and within the group there is an opportunity to discover that their peers have problems that they thought were unique to themselves, (c) acquiring a deeper sense of altruism, (d) correcting maladaptive patterns acquired in the primary family group, (e) the acquisition of social skills, (f) the imitation of prosocial behaviour, (g) interpersonal learning, (h) group cohesiveness, (i) catharsis, which essentially consists of allowing children to discharge their emotions within overall limits, (j) existential factors, which include the notion that life is at times unfair and unjust and that perhaps there is ultimately no escape from some of the hurt of life experiences, and (k) that group members must ultimately come to take responsibility for the way in which they live their own lives.

Other writers identify those factors that are of importance to the organisation and the functioning of groups. For instance, Bloch and Crouch point out that the qualities of the group make a contribution, such as the group's goals, size, composition, duration, context, and stages of development (see section on composition of groups).[21]

Some advantages of psychotherapy groups

(1) Unlike adults in therapy, children are dependent on others for attendance at therapy sessions. Thus there are many children who would not attend as outpatients for regular psychotherapy because their families are unwilling or unable to provide the necessary support. However, it is possible for group psychotherapy to be "taken to the child" in other settings, such as those enumerated below.

(2) Psychotherapy groups can be run in many settings that may not easily provide the conditions necessary for individual psychotherapeutic work—for example in children's homes, ordinary schools, and remand homes.[15] For instance, it has proved possible to run groups in what might be considered the rather unpromising circumstances of normal junior and even senior schools by restructuring the environment available, setting sensible limits, and working within timetable constraints.[4]

(3) Some parents are unable to tolerate the suggestion that their child needs therapeutic help because they perceive this as singling out their child, and for them an offer of group psychotherapy is often less threatening.

(4) When assessment indicates that group psychotherapy is the best treatment then it may be a more economic use of the therapist's time.

(5) Many of the children, but particularly adolescents, referred for psychotherapeutic help suffer a sense of loneliness and isolation. For them a psychotherapy group offers a safe, supportive, empathic setting where boundaries and limits are determined by the therapist and where there is an opportunity for immediate acceptance, first by the therapist or therapists and then by the other group members. For many children it is their first experience of becoming an important part of the life of a peer group and an opportunity, in a safe setting, of learning how to make friends.

(6) Within the group the children are each enabled to see the consequences of their own behaviour and to see the impact of the behaviour of others on themselves. Thus because the group experience is shared children have an opportunity to see not only the consequences of their own projections, but also how they may be vulnerable to the projections of others. For example, the bullied child may be helped to see that he or she is subtly provoking others to bully and how and why they do so.

(7) Being in the company of children with different personal-

> ## Box 1—Advantages of psychotherapy groups
> - Can be undertaken in many settings which may not easily provide the necessary conditions for individual psychotherapy—for example, ordinary schools
> - May be less threatening than individual treatment for those parents who find it hard to bear the notion that their child needs therapeutic help
> - Can be a more economic use of therapist time
> - Especially helpful to promote socialisation in children and adolescents
> - Can help children see and reflect on the impact of their behaviour on others
> - May enable the child to rediscover some of his or her own psychological weaknesses and strengths by observing the behaviour of others
> - Allows the exploration of relationships, different models of behaviour, and perspectives on situations.

ities, and seeing their weaknesses and strengths, enables the child to rediscover aspects of himself or herself that have been suppressed and to value the positive qualities she or he already has, thus enhancing a feeling of self worth.

(8) The group facilitates the exploration of several relationships and offers different models of behaviour and different perspectives on situations. This is particularly helpful for many deprived children, and for all children who have little capacity for reflection at the time of referral. Similarly, with older children or even those who are relatively adolescent, group processes and the appreciation that personal problems are not unique may facilitate self disclosure.

(9) Each member of the group will acquire a memory of all the events that have an important impact on the life of the group. This is particularly helpful for those children who have been traumatised psychologically by their own life experiences and seem able to retain or learn little. In individual therapy, experiences and events can be denied and responsibility refused, but in the group it is more difficult over time to deny experiences that the group insists have occurred.

(10) It is hoped that positive group experiences will carry over into settings outside the group, such as the family and the school— indeed there is some empirical evidence that group therapy in schools using non-directive principles[3] gives rise to improvement in behaviour in both the classroom and the home.[4]

Who can run psychodynamic psychotherapy groups?

Group psychotherapy can be undertaken by a wide range of professionals whose basic training has enabled them to observe, listen to, and communicate with children about their feelings, to clarify issues, and to help them to understand the meaning of their interactions. However, it is mandatory for the above basic training to be complemented by further training, which includes regular supervision provided by clinicians experienced in psychodynamic group approaches. It is also possible for those with training and experience to work with those who wish to learn, by functioning as cotherapists. Cotherapy provides an important opportunity for cross disciplinary work; for example, a child psychotherapist or a child psychiatrist with appropriate training might work with a special teacher, a nurse, or a paediatrician.

Composition of groups

TYPES OF GROUPS

Settings, age, and sex

Groups are conducted in many settings, with the nature of the group often determined by the nature of the setting where children may congregate (nursery, school, special educational, or residential settings). Here a mixed group of children share a setting, such as a school, and therefore have some knowledge of each other before and outside the group setting. In other cases they are brought together because of common behavioral problems (clinics, hospital units, or other units for troubled children); and age (children or adolescents). Thus groups can focus on a particular age group or sex group (for example, abused girls) or mixed sex groups.

Families or siblings

If several children in a family are all felt to be in need of help, family therapy may be the treatment of choice; however, some parents may refuse to discuss difficulties with their children present. One solution would be to see the siblings together, which facilitates the exploration of the ways in which they see not only each other but also the parent or parents.[12 22 23] Similarly, when there is a shared traumatic event, such as the sudden death of a parent, with its consequent serious distress then working with the siblings as a group could be the initial treatment of choice.

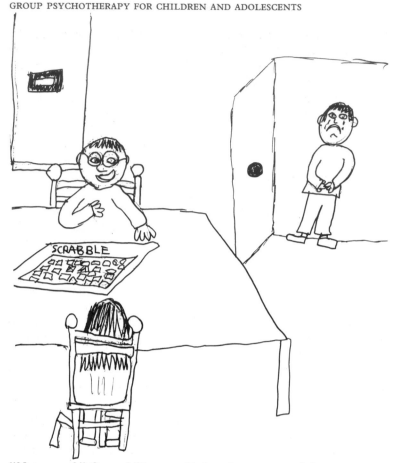

"Not wanted." Some children need help to become part of the peer group

Other groups

In other groups the focus may be children who are not in the same family but who may have been exposed to a similar traumatising experience, such as sexual abuse, or who share in a traumatic event, such as a fire or a disaster. These children may have experienced no major psychological difficulties before the event, and this constitutes an opportunity to help the children to work through and to cope with the experience. These groups differ from other groups in that they can usefully be restricted to brief focal work, needing perhaps as few as six sessions.

There is not wide agreement about the composition of groups: some workers prefer to address a heterogeneity of problems within the same group (mixed group), whereas others focus on similar traumas or disorders. Thus, some workers will group together sexually abused children or anorexic young people. Those preferring to use a heterogeneity model would argue that even sexually abused children need to have other aspects of their life experiences understood, and to have the opportunity to have their individual strengths and vulnerabilities attended to. Such children sometimes complain that a group for sexually abused children can make them feel like a "sex abuse case" only and may deprive them of their individuality, whereas in a mixed group the sexually abused child can choose when it is the experience of the abuse that she or he wishes to be addressed and when he or she is to be allowed to be seen as a child with other strengths and preoccupations; here, the child sets the agenda. Others would argue that for some children a homogeneous group is a safe and reliable setting for sexual abuse experiences to emerge and be explored.

In summary, though there is a consensus that the composition of the group is critical to its success or failure, some argue for homogeneity of disordered behaviour and others see "mix" as the essential element including a sex mix. Those advocating mix stress that when selecting children for a group careful thought should be given to the balance of problems and personalities.[14 15] For example, including an excess of children described as violent or acting out would be unlikely to allow for therapeutic work to be done, as the leaders would be occupied simply in preventing disasters. Similarly, a group of very timid children together is likely to become flat in its emotional atmosphere. A wide range of personalities and presenting problems increases the possibility of identification for the children within the group.

SIZE OF GROUPS

Group psychotherapy with children and young adolescents encompasses two distinct sub groups—those who are about 5–11 years old and those about 11–15 years old. Many children are sensitive about the issue of age and, once at secondary school, may see themselves as beyond childish things, even if this may not in reality be reflected by their developmental level; they can be deeply worried by being grouped with "children". Younger children's groups are most successful when composed of four or five children. Some group therapists opt for five to allow for potential drop outs. However, this is the largest number that children aged up to 11 can relate to therapeutically and often the most that can be contained, as children of this age are prone to acting out and need to be kept safe. Adolescents need a larger group, six to nine young people, for two main reasons: firstly, absenteeism is not uncommon and it is wise to expect that not all members will arrive for each session: secondly, they sometimes find a smaller group too intimate.

Organisation and setting

To run a psychotherapy group successfully a suitable setting, and equipment for younger children, need to be available. For example, the room needs to be "safe" and not, for example, subject to interruption from outside during the sessions; any potential dangers to children need to be minimised (for instance, by having windows that are securely fastened); the room should be reasonably near a toilet; and appropriate play material should be available, which potentially encourages group activities. The duration of sessions should be fixed beforehand and firmly adhered to—an hour for the 5–11 year olds and an hour and a quarter for young adolescents. Holiday arrangements should be agreed before the onset of the group. It is important to meet and prepare each child individually before the group sessions begin, so that they are aware of expectations of them throughout the duration of the group's life and of the nature of the therapy; this can lead to improved attendance.[24]

The setting also refers to the atmosphere, created by the therapist or cotherapist, within which therapeutic work can take place. To this end, at the first meeting a group therapist should provide structure and guidance, introducing the children to each other, explaining about the length of the sessions, and suggesting minimal rules. This approach is commonly used in institutional settings for children with antisocial behaviour. Others consider it important for children without major antisocial behaviour to have the opportunity to discover any rules, and that these are likely to be minimal—restricted only to limiting behaviour that would physically damage other children, the room, or the leaders or behaviour that might unduly hurt another child's feelings.[3]

Who can benefit? What are the contraindications?

Group therapy was previously thought to be indicated for those children and adolescents who could not tolerate or be accommodated by individual therapy. However, this is no longer seen as correct as clinical experience has shown that children with a wide range of problems can make use of group therapy, provided that careful consideration is given to the composition of the groups. Children whose difficulties with their peers predominate often seem ideal candidates for a group.[4 15 25] In paediatric settings, for example, group therapy has been used with children in hospital for chronic illness or who present with homogeneous and focused problems such as obesity.[26] Nevertheless, individual psychotherapy, where available, might commonly be the treatment of choice. Decisions about whether individual or group therapy should be used, where both are available, will be determined by assessing the child and local resources.

Different theorists offer different suggestions why some subjects should be excluded: for instance, Aveline argues (for adults) that those who are brain damaged, psychologically fragile, or who deny the psychological basis of their difficulties are not yet able to benefit from group therapy and need the intimacy of the one to one therapeutic relationship and should be excluded;[27] however (with children) skilled therapists find that they can include a wider mix of disorders.[15]

The role of the therapist

LEADERSHIP

Children and young adolescent groups can be led by a single leader. When there are cotherapists for a group it is helpful (but not essential) to have a male and a female therapist; but it is essential that there is a basic respect and liking between these therapists.[15] The role of the therapist or therapists in a children's therapy group differs from that in an adult therapy group, in that in children's groups dependency on the leader is appropriate—for instance, the leader may have to protect certain children; it is acknowledged that such dependency is developmentally healthy.[15] Thus, the therapist (or cotherapist) must demonstrate a capacity to contain and protect all the members of the group. Hence the group therapist has to forge a therapeutic alliance that is appropriate to their age and aimed at helping the group to appreciate that one of their tasks is to be aware of painful thoughts and feelings and how to share and cope with them.[28] The impact of the group on the therapist or therapists (and vice versa) should never be underestimated—for instance, where there are cotherapists the group may exaggerate what they perceive to be the individual qualities of each therapist, and this could lead to a schism between therapists.[15]

THERAPEUTIC BOUNDARIES

As previously indicated, the children must be contained, not only within the physical space provided by the room, but they also need to be kept in mind (psychologically) by the therapists. It follows from this that it is essential to know what every member of the group is doing at any one time, and this is the skill that most group therapists find the most difficult to develop within the often hurly-burly atmosphere of the group. When the boundaries of the room are firmly kept to and the adults also contain the group firmly in the mind, then it is possible to allow considerable freedom of behaviour, wishes, and impulses within this framework. Without this structure the therapy cannot take place.

EQUALITY, ACCEPTANCE, AND RESPECT

The experience of equality is established by the therapist by a concrete demonstration that each individual has equal right of access to the therapist. In time, equality comes to be understood as not necessarily equivalent to the same amount of time with or from the leader within any one session. Equality is emphasised by the therapist noticing, for example, that one child is not asking for time or attention and bringing this to the attention of that child and also limiting any child who may be in danger of monopolising the leader. As long as this is done by way of observation and not criticism it will also facilitate the experience of equality. Acceptance within the group means accepting each individual child as he or she is when first joining the group, without criticism, but rather with the aim of understanding that child and his or her problems. However, acceptance does not mean putting up with intolerable behaviour. An accepting atmosphere within the group soon seems to become infectious, with the children themselves rapidly developing a capacity to tolerate behaviour that they previously found unacceptable. Acceptance is often followed by a sense of trust and group cohesion.

Stated simply, the therapist strives to create a warm, accepting atmosphere that is friendly to the development of ideas and the exploration of relationships. The therapist should also strive to be alert to any expression of a wish to change in a child, or curiosity by a child about their own behaviour. Each child is respected as the person he or she is and this attitude is encouraged in the other

---

Box 2—Treatment strategies in group therapy

- Creation of a warm, accepting atmosphere, friendly to the development of ideas and exploration of relationships
- Principles of equality, acceptance, and respect
- Leader importance in:
  - (a) containing and protecting members of the group
  - (b) forging a therapeutic alliance that is age appropriate
  - (c) providing the therapeutic boundaries
  - (d) providing support and encouragement, allowing the development of new relationships, and seeking to understand those factors in each child that hinder this.

---

children in the group. The therapists are there to support, encourage, and allow the development of new relationships and to try to understand the factors in each child that hinder this.

Efficacy and prognosis

INTRODUCTION

Until the early 1980s there were only a few studies of group therapy with children that used non-directive techniques focusing on improving academic performance, peer relationships, or behaviour. Unfortunately, many of the early studies provided few details of the therapy process, beyond a label such as "non-directive" or "didactic". Often there were serious methodological limitations with these studies. Nevertheless, there was a trend for the more substantial studies to focus on solving academic issues.

Those studies, which were of reasonable scientific rigour, gave rise to a diversity of outcome.[29 30 31] For instance, some group therapy endeavours have been aimed at intelligence and achievements, but systematic research has shown that such therapy can influence socialisation and behaviour more readily than cognition.[4 32] Such studies often lead to an improvement on measures reflecting the views of peers (sociometric measures) and those studies that focused on difficult behaviour reported by the teachers also tended to give positive results.[33 34] Finally, several studies have been undertaken that focused on improving children's self concept, and these almost always gave positive results.[35 36] An important follow up study of a large series of sexually abused children suggests that group forms of therapy are effective.[37] Though this gives cause for optimism, there is equally cause for caution, both because the drop out rate was high and (as it was an uncontrolled study) there was no way of estimating the extent of the effect of natural reparative processes.

THE NEWCASTLE PROGRAMMES

Unfortunately, many of the previously published studies were reduced in value because of serious problems of small sample size, high rates of drop out, questionable statistical analysis and, often, inadequate measures. Nevertheless, despite these limitations, in many cases the results were encouraging. The largest and most systematic of the studies was that undertaken by the Newcastle school (see also chapter 14).[38 39] The aim of that study was the prevention and treatment of psychiatric disturbance reflecting neurotic and antisocial behaviour presenting in the school setting and it involved 7–8 year olds and 11–12 year olds. The children in these studies were identified with a multiple criterion screen, which covered behaviour and sociometric functioning.

Basic philosophy

The group therapies were based originally on the philosophy developed by Rogers.[40] The adaptation of the group therapy technique to younger children was influenced by the work of Axline in the USA,[2] especially her eight principles that could be followed in practical play therapy. These include (a) the development of a warm, friendly relationship with the child; (b) accepting the child as he or she is; (c) engendering a sense of permissiveness in the relationship; (d) being alert to the expression of feelings in the child; (e) maintaining a deep respect for the child's ability to solve his or her own problems; (f) having a non-directive attitude; (g) exerting no sense of pressure; and finally (h) confining limit setting to those boundaries that are necessary to maintain the therapy in the real world. The above therapeutic policy allowed the children to reflect their feelings through play in groups. Nevertheless, it was necessary to establish some limit setting to allow the groups to function in the complex environment of the school, while at the same time strengthening internal controls of some of the more impulsive children.[13] Similar groups were run in secondary schools.

Long term follow up studies were undertaken some 30–66 months after the start of the treatment programme. Non-treated control groups were used to establish base rates of moderately good and good outcomes, which occurred in under half the control subjects; but good outcome occurred in about three quarters of the subjects of group therapy.

Treatment specificity

Another attractive theme in psychotherapy research is that different types of disorders respond to different kinds of psychotherapy. These kinds of treatment specificity, which are so important in adult disorders, do not appear to be supported by the work described above (the Newcastle studies) with children and adolescents, where the effects of group therapy were compared with other forms of psychotherapy. There was no consistent evidence of specificity, such as a better response of children with conduct or neurotic disorders to different treatment or management programmes such as behaviour modification or group therapy; where treatment was effective, it proved to be more so for neurotic disorders and less so for conduct disorders, but there was no particular form of psychotherapy that was more effective for one or other disorder.

Dimension of time—long term follow up and "sleeper effects"

It is important to try to locate beneficial changes within a time frame. It is commonly believed that patients respond gradually to psychotherapeutic help, with a maximum response being achieved by the end of treatment, after which patients may reach a plateau or, with the cessation of therapeutic support, the effects of treatment may begin to dissipate. In the Newcastle studies, when examining outcomes over time, it was intriguing to find that treatment effects continued to increase some 18 months or so after the end of treatment. The failure of the controls to catch up by the end of the follow up period also suggests that positive processes had been set in motion by the therapy.

Of particular importance is the subject of long term follow up. As mentioned, the findings from the Newcastle studies suggest that even relatively brief group therapy may have effects long after termination of treatment, and these may not be detected unless provision is made for long term follow up. In these school based treatment studies it seemed that it was the type (for example, relatively brief group therapy) rather than the duration of treatment (for example, long term casework with parents) that was a critical factor in intervention. However, this may not be true for more seriously disturbed children in either hospital based or clinical settings.

The concept of "sleeper effects", that is delayed effects of therapy, and their possible impact on the results of therapy, including group therapy, holds considerable fascination for the therapist and researcher alike. Whereas there is evidence that assessments at the end of treatment and at short term follow up give rise to no major differences between group therapy subjects and controls, such differences proved to be substantial at long term follow up; thus, it would seem that improvement continues after therapy has ceased. The mechanisms behind this remain unknown.[41] Although measurement of these delayed effects poses no problems, the mechanism of the psychological processes that precede the delayed effects is not easy to elucidate. One possible explanation is that positive social interactions within a therapy group may lead to a strengthening of relationships with peers, which may be reinforced by subsequent further contacts with these peers outside the therapy groups. Another possibility is that the child may acquire a new set of skills through group interactional experiences that are not useful immediately, but subsequently become so; for instance, they may help to prepare children to cope with later stressful experiences. Alternatively, there may be subtle shifts in personality that, through feedback mechanisms, give rise to demonstrable changes in behaviour.

Conclusion

Some workers report an immediate response to some forms of group therapy. Even when this does not occur, however, whatever the mechanism involved, the therapist should not be deterred by lack of evidence of immediate or even short term overt behavioural changes with seriously disturbed children but should check for the presence of longer term, more durable effects in due course.

According to Yalom,[42] the child constructs an individual inner world that can be reconstructed through interactions with others. The inner world refers to the notion that each of us has an imaginative life, or world of the mind, in which there is an alive continuing relationship between all the important figures, particularly parent figures, and experiences of the external world. Furthermore, the inner and outer worlds are equally real and important to the child. The crucial influences are the therapist's expectations of the children and also the modification of the children's perception of themselves. Group therapy will enable those in a group to understand how other people function and how their own inner assumptions powerfully determine the pattern of subsequent interactions.[27]

1 Slavson SR. *An introduction to group therapy.* New York: International Universities Press, 1943.
2 Axline VM. *Play therapy.* Boston: Houghton Mifflin, 1947.
3 Rogers CR. *Client-centred therapy.* Boston: Houghton Mifflin, 1952.
4 Kolvin I, Garside RF, Nicol AR, Macmillan A, Wolstenholme F, Leitch IM. *Help starts here. The maladjusted child in the ordinary school.* London and New York: Tavistock Publications, 1981.
5 Klein M. *Contributions to psychoanalysis.* London: Hogarth Press and Institute of Psychoanalysis, 1921–45.
6 Klein M. *Envy and gratitude* and other works. London: Hogarth Press and Institute of Psychoanalysis, 1946–63.
7 Klein M. *Our adult world and its roots in infancy.* London: Tavistock Publications, 1961.
8 Klein M. *The psychoanalysis of children.* London: Hogarth Press and Institute of Psychoanalysis, 1932.
9 Bion WR. Advances in group and individual therapy. In: JC Flugel, ed. *International Congress on Mental Health. Proceedings of the International Conference on Medical Psychotherapy.* London: HK Lewis, 1948;3:106–10.
10 Bion WR. *Experiences in groups.* London: Tavistock Publications, 1961.
11 Reid S. Group work with children in schools. In: M Fox, L Kennedy, eds. *Proceedings of the 1991 Conference for Education. Psychology in Training.* Tavistock Occasional Papers, 1991.
12 Reid S. *A psychoanalytic approach to group psychotherapy with children.* London: 1993 (in press).
13 Ginott H. *Group psychotherapy with children.* New York: McGraw-Hill, 1961.
14 Reid S, Fry, E, Rhode M. Working with small groups of children in primary schools. In: Daws D. Boston M, eds. *The child psychotherapist.* London: Karnac, 1988: 31 63.
15 Reid S. The use of groups for therapeutic interventions. In: Thacker VJ, ed. *Prevention and intervention. Working with groups.* Division of Educational and Child Psychology, British Psychological Society, occasional papers, 1987; 3 and 4: 171–9.
16 Winnicott DW. *Playing and reality.* London: Tavistock, 1971.
17 Freud S. *Introductory lectures in psychoanalysis.* London: Allen and Unwin, 1922.
18 Sherrif M, Sherrif CW. *Social psychology* New York: Harper and Row, 1969.
19 Whitaker DS, Lieberman MA. *Psychotherapy through the group process.* London: Tavistock, 1965.
20 Yalom ID. *The theory and practice of group psychotherapy.* 2nd ed. New York: Basic Books, 1975.
21 Bloch S, Crouch E. *Therapeutic factors in group psychotherapy.* Oxford: Oxford University Press, 1985.
22 Hammond JM. Loss of the family unit: counselling groups to help kids. *Personnel and Guidance* 1981;59:392–4.
23 Schaefer CE, Johnson L, Wherry JN. *Group therapies for children and youth.* San Francisco and London: Jossey Bass, 1982.
24 Kendall PC, Zupan BA. Individual versus group applications of cognitive-behavioral self-control procedures with children. *Behavior Therapy* 1981;12:344–59.
25 Hargrave GE, Hargrave ML. A peer group socialization therapy program in the school: an outcome investigation. *Psychotherapy in the Schools* 1979;16:546–50.

26 Brownell KD, Kelman JH, Stukard AJ. Treatment of obese children with and without their mothers: changes in weight and blood pressure. *Pediatrics* 1983;**71**:515–23.
27 Aveline M. *From medicine to psychotherapy*. London: Whurr Publishers, 1992.
28 Cramer-Azuma FJ. Group psychotherapy for children and adolescents. In: Melvin Lewis, ed. *Child and adolescent psychiatry. A comprehensive textbook.* Baltimore: Williams & Wilkins, 1987.
29 Bevins SMC. A comparison of the effectiveness of individual and group counselling in the improvement of social adjustment of 5th and 6th grade children. *Dissertation Abstracts International* 1970;**30A**:5277 (abstract).
30 Schiffer M. *The therapeutic play group*. London: Allen and Unwin, 1971.
31 Thombs MR, Muro JJ. Group counselling and the sociometric status of second grade children. *Elementary School Guidance and Counselling* 1973;**7**:194–7.
32 McGuire J, Earls F. Prevention of psychiatric disorders in early childhood. *J Child Psychol Psychiatry* 1991;**33**:129–54.
33 Barcai A, Robinson EH. Conventional group therapy with preadolescent children. *Int J Group Psychother* 1969;**19**:334–45.
34 Hubbert AK. Effect of group counselling and behaviour modification on attentive behaviour of first grade students. *Dissertation Abstracts International* 1970;**30A**:3727 (abstract).
35 Hugo MJ. The effects of group counselling on self-concept and behaviour of elementary school children. *Dissertation Abstracts International* 1970;**30A**:3728 (abstract).
36 Mann PH, Barber JD, Jacobson MD. The effect of group counselling on educable mentally retarded boys' self-concepts. *Except Child* 1969;**35**:354–66.
37 Bentovim A, Boston P, Van Elburg A. Child sexual abuse—children and families referred to a treatment project and the effects of intervention. *BMJ* 1987;**295**:1453–7.
38 Nicol AR, Parker J. Playgroup therapy in the junior school. I. Method and general problems. *British Journal of Guidance and Counselling* 1981;**9**:86–93.
39 Parker J, Nicol AR. Playgroup therapy in the junior school. II. The therapy process. *British Journal of Guidance and Counselling* 1981;**9**:202–6.
40 Hall CS, Lindzey G. *Theories of personality*. New York: Wiley, 1970.
41 Bell V, Lyne S, Kolvin I. Play group therapy: processes and patterns and delayed effects. In: MH Schmidt, H Remschmidt, eds. *Needs and prospects of child and adolescent psychiatry*. Stuttgart: Hogrefe and Huber, 1989.
42 Yalom ID. *The theory and practice of group psychotherapy*. 3rd ed. New York: Basic Books, 1985.

7. Drug treatment

Michael Prendergast

There is general agreement that psychoactive drugs should only be given as part of an overall treatment plan, which will often include other treatment methods described in this book. It might be thought there would also be general agreement that the use of psychoactive drugs should be informed by empirical findings, but there are such large differences in prescribing practice between clinicians and between countries that other factors must be relevant. Stimulant drugs are probably the best investigated and best understood psychoactive drugs in use in childhood and yet they are seldom prescribed in Britain, where drugs are frequently used to treat sleep problems and nocturnal enuresis.[1][2] Both of these conditions are more appropriately managed with behavioural methods. Some severe psychiatric problems are unusual and little researched in childhood or adolescence. One can appeal to the adult literature for guidance on drug treatment in these cases. Child psychiatry publications contain several reviews of pharmacotherapy which differ in emphasis and which are helpful in whole or in part.[3-7]

There is still quite a gap between our knowledge of what drugs can do biochemically and why they make some problems better. Most psychoactive drugs affect more than one neurotransmitter system,[8] so this account leaves neurotransmitters aside and matches operationally defined syndromes with drugs believed to alter target symptoms within these syndromes.

Sleep problems

Difficulty in settling, "midnight intruder", and dawn rising are common sleep problems in the toddler years and respond well to behavioural methods, which are the treatment of choice.[9] Prescription of hypnotics to children is contraindicated by the *British National Formulary*[10]; despite this, their use is widespread.[1] Trimeprazine works well in the short term[11] and may be used in a crisis, for example, when parents are severely sleep deprived themselves. Tolerance develops rapidly and if the response is to increase the dose the child may become zombie-like and drool throughout the day. Data sheets for trimeprazine now contain an expanded section on the risk of tardive dyskinesia, which is another reason for caution. Chloral is an alternative for short term use. Benzodiazepines are best avoided in childhood because of their behavioural toxicity.

Occasional nightmares are common and can usually be related to a frightening experience. If frequent they should be psychologically investigated. Night terrors, sleep walking, and sleep talking are parasomnias and often respond to explanation and reassurance.[12] When they are frequent and occur at a predictable time of the night, they can sometimes be controlled by pre-emptive waking.[13] Drug treatment is rarely necessary. Low dose benzodiazepines have been used and there are reports of successful use of both imipramine[14] and carbamazepine,[15] which may be preferred.

Narcolepsy and other hypersomnias are seldom diagnosed in childhood. Psychostimulants, for example, methylphenidate or dexamphetamine, and more recently mazindol,[16] are favoured in the adult literature. Clomipramine may reduce the frequency of narcoleptic attacks and of cataplexy, which is loss of tone without loss of consciousness.[12] Dietary tyrosine supplements have been found helpful in reducing hypersomnia in adults in some hands[17] but not in others.[18] Quantitative serum tyrosine monitoring is prudent in childhood.

Confusion and delirium

Confusion and delirium are medical emergencies and this is the first line of management. Fever or other signs may point to a medical cause and non-convulsive status epilepticus is one of many conditions that must be considered. Drugs may be responsible, whether medically prescribed or illicitly obtained, through idiosyncratic reaction or overdose.

When a drug is responsible for the reaction it should be withdrawn if possible. Disorientation and behaviour disturbance are often more prominent at night, and chloral is effective if only night sedation is required.

Where behaviour disturbance is jeopardising treatment, the short term use of chlorpromazine is recommended, in doses sufficient to confine the child to bed, combined with adequate illumination and sensitive nursing care. Such reactions are usually shortlived.

Children with dementing illnesses associated with behavioural problems may rarely require chronic sedation, chlorpromazine or thioridazine, for example, which should be prescribed in the lowest dose effective and in higher dose at night if night time sedation is also required. The oral route is preferred as intramuscular injections may be interpreted as attacks. Where tablets are not tolerated and when thioridazine is chosen, the suspension should be used as the liquid is extremely unpalatable.

Schizophrenia, hallucinations, and neuroleptic drugs

Schizophrenia of adult type is rare in prepubertal children, although it becomes more common in adolescence. Its management is a specialist matter and will often involve inpatient treatment in a dedicated unit. An underlying physical disorder should always be sought. Treatment is symptomatic and based on the symptoms present at the time.

As drug treatment hinges on neuroleptics with their attendant long term risk of tardive dyskinesia, non-drug alternatives can and perhaps should be tried where appropriate, although it is recognised that most units do not do this.

Auditory hallucinations may respond to an ear plug.[19] It should be placed in the more impaired ear where there is a difference, and when the patient will tolerate it. Visual hallucinations are usually paroxysmal, and distorting spectacles interfere with them if the patient can be persuaded to sit down and use them. Both these types of hallucinations can occur in plain consciousness in the absence of psychosis.[20 21] In these circumstances, compliance with the treatments suggested above may be easier to obtain.

The drug treatment of children and adolescents with schizophrenia is little researched, and practice is based on analogy with the adult literature.

It is important to appreciate the huge differences in potency between neuroleptics. A dose of 100 mg of chlorpromazine is equivalent to: 100 mg of thioridazine, 5 mg of trifluoperazine, only 2 mg of haloperidol, only 2 mg of pimozide, but 200 mg of sulpiride, and 40 mg of clozapine. In general, the more potent neuroleptics carry a greater risk of extrapyramidal side effects and the less potent neuroleptics are more sedative, but still have extrapyramidal side effects. Depending on the degree of disturbance at presentation, sedation may be the first priority. Otherwise, a period of drug free inpatient observation by experienced staff is preferable and may be all that is required in some brief psychotic episodes.

Subsequent management in those requiring medication will comprise a systematic trial of several weeks of a drug from each of the various groups, given individually according to tolerance. Typical representatives would be chlorpromazine, thioridazine, sulpiride, and haloperidol. Depot neuroleptics are usually avoided until a stable response has been obtained, if they are to be used at all.

Unfortunately, a therapeutic margin between symptom relief and side effects can be hard to find in the prepubertal patient.[22] Clozapine offers hope for treatment resistant patients but it is only licensed for use in children older than 12 years subject to compliance with an expensive monitoring procedure to guard against agranulocytosis.[23]

Drug treatment affects mainly the positive symptoms of hallucinations and delusions. It has very little effect on the negative motivationless state that some patients are left with. Ciompi has drawn attention to the various patterns of schizophrenic illness.[24] Only some forms imply "medication for life". Once control is achieved, a decision must be made whether to try the patient with a diminished drug dosage while still in hospital, or after safe return home. The issue of continued treatment should be kept under continual review. Antiparkinsonian agents are not prescribed routinely but are given only if parkinsonian side effects occur.

Patient and parents must be warned of the possibility of writhing, dystonic movements of the face and body, and oculogyric crisis in the first few days of treatment with neuroleptics and of parkinsonian symptoms of tremor, rigidity, akinesia, and salivation in the succeeding weeks. All of these symptoms respond to antiparkinsonian agents or medication reduction. Acute dystonic reactions are distressing and constitute medical emergencies. Parents of children who are managed as outpatients may be given a few procyclidine tablets or equivalent to use, if required, pending attendance at a casualty department. Intramuscular injection of an antiparkinsonian drug will bring more immediate relief.

Some patients experience akathisia, an unpleasant restless agitation, usually within the first two months of starting a neuroleptic. It can be difficult to treat without drug reduction. Adult work

Typical onset intervals for neuroleptic induced extrapyramidal disorders

Acute dystonias (oculogyric crisis, etc)	Within hours to 7 days
Akathisia	Within hours to 2 months
Parkinsonism (akinesia/rigidity/tremor)	Within first month
Tardive dyskinesia	Usually after 3 months
Tardive akathisia	Usually after months
Tardive dystonia	3 Days to 11 years
Neuroleptic malignant syndrome	At any time.

indicates that akathisia is relatively resistant to antiparkinsonian drugs but propranolol may be helpful. Clonazepam has been found to be effective in some adolescent cases.[25]

More seriously, neuroleptic malignant syndrome may present at any time.[26] In its florid state it is characterised by fever, fluctuating consciousness, autonomic instability, increased tone, and raised serum creatine kinase. Formes frustes occur and fever or raised enzymes may be lacking. It is a potentially lethal condition. Neuroleptics must be stopped at once. Symptoms may take a week or more to respond but longer if the patient has taken a depot neuroleptic.

Dantrolene and bromocriptine have been used but the essence of treatment is attention to fluid balance and cardiorespiratory support in a medical setting.

Tardive dyskinesia is an important long term risk of neuroleptic treatment. It may be transient and appear as a withdrawal dyskinesia lasting from days to several months, or it may be persistent. In tardive dyskinesia irregular choreoathetoid movements occur predominantly in the buccal-lingual musculature and at the distal extremities. It is not uncommon in children exposed to neuroleptic, 22% in one series.[27] Mentally retarded patients are at greater risk and also at greater risk of being given neuroleptic treatment. Tardive dystonia is a more malignant variant characterised by sustained contraction of skeletal musculature, manifest as, for example, sustained tongue protrusion, disabling posturing, stridor from laryngospasm, and dysarthria.[7 28] In addition, Gualtieri has described a late onset behavioural equivalent of tardive dyskinesia that he terms tardive akathisia with dysphoria and motor restlessness.[7]

All these conditions are difficult to treat beyond withdrawal of neuroleptics and waiting. They may be irreversible but remission rates in children are fortunately higher than in adults.[6 7 27]

Non-extrapyramidal side effects of neuroleptics include gynaecomastia, galactorrhoea, amenorrhoea, weight gain, and jaundice. Chlorpromazine is particularly associated with photosensitive reactions, and thioridazine in high dose with a pigmentary retinopathy.

Hypomania and bipolar illness

Hypomania is characterised by elevated mood, excitement and irritability, pressure of talk and flight of ideas, which are often grandoise. Teenagers are disinhibited and sleep little. Mania is a more florid version of the same. It is rare, even reportable before the teenage years.[29] In the acute phase, sedation with a major tranquilliser and hospital admission may be required. Hypomanic episodes may be recurrent, or more usually part of a bipolar illness. Children and teenagers with bipolar disorders have recurrent episodes of severe depression and hypomania. Lithium carbonate is the treatment of choice.[6 30] Because of differences in bioavailability, it is important to choose a preparation and stay with it.

Sustained release lithium carbonate can be given twice a day and blood concentrations are monitored in the steady state, 12 hours after the previous dose. In practice this means about five days after the last dose increase. Target serum concentrations are usually within the range of 0·6–1·0 mmol/l. When control is obtained, measurements are repeated every six weeks or so and also thyroid function tests and tests of renal function are performed—less frequently but more often if there is cause for concern. Fluid loss through vomiting, diarrhoea, and sweating in hot weather can all cause toxicity that is characterised by diarrhoea, vomiting, tremor, ataxia, dysarthria, and muscular weakness progressing to cardiac arrhythmia, stupor, and death if lithium is continued. Less severe side effects include polydipsia, polyuria, weight gain, and thyroid dysfunction. Previous worries about nephrotoxicity seem to have been exaggerated.[31]

In rapid cycling bipolar illnesses there are three or more occurrences within a year. Sometimes there may be several mood swings within a week. Carbamazepine can be used as an alternative to lithium carbonate in unresponsive patients and as a treatment of choice in rapid cycling patients,[32] as can sodium valproate.[32a]

Dosages are the same as in the treatment of epilepsy, and the sustained release carbamazepine preparation is preferred.

Depression

Depression of adult type is increasingly recognised in childhood. In the past it was probably included in the category of emotional disorders without further inquiry.

When depression is suspected, the child must be interviewed alone and suicidal ideas inquired after. A decision should be made about whether referral for inpatient treatment is required. Although child psychiatrists use antidepressants to treat the more serious depressions,[2] evidence from double blind trials to support this practice is lacking so far and the issue is unresolved. There is little experience with the new antidepressants.[32b]

Typically, amitriptyline is used for its sedative effect in the agitated patient and imipramine is used for its more stimulant effect in the patient who has slowed up. Patients and parents should be warned about the early appearance and resolution of the anticholinergic effects of dry mouth, constipation, and blurred vision. These are not usually problematic if the drug is introduced slowly. Children seem to require 75–100 mg daily on average and starting at 25 mg at night, the dose can be increased by a similar increment every three days or so.

The antidepressant effect is not usually obtained before about 10 days of treatment at the appropriate dose. In responders to treatment antidepressants are usually continued for about three months after response is obtained. I do not usually begin withdrawal of drugs at critical times, for example, at the start of the new school year. Intersubject variation in absorption of imipramine is considerable, and monitoring of blood concentrations is recommended when this tricyclic is used. Puig-Antich et al have suggested that a total plasma concentration of 150 µg/l (imipramine and desipramine) is necessary for therapeutic effect.[33] Serial electrocardiographic (ECG) records are recommended if high doses of imipramine are needed to achieve this.[6] Clearly, parents must understand the need to supervise the taking of tablets and to keep them away from the patient and younger siblings. Childproof containers are essential.[34]

Sleep deprivation or deprivation of rapid eye movement sleep as treatments for depression have yielded inconsistent results but may offer a treatment alternative for antidepressant resistant patients.[35][36]

Very severe depressive illness unresponsive to antidepressants, depressive stupor, and catatonic stupor are rare indications for electroconvulsive treatment. It should not be undertaken without further supportive consultant opinions, perhaps from colleagues in adolescent psychiatry and adult psychiatry, in addition to the usual thorough discussion with patient and parents. The great advantage of electroconvulsive treatment is rapid relief when it is successful.[37]

Obsessive compulsive disorders and trichotillomania

The manifestations of obsessive compulsive disorder include repetitious checking and other rituals and compulsions which often involve the whole family. Children who are severely handicapped by these symptoms may require inpatient treatment.

Behavioural management has a role but it is less powerful in this condition than was originally thought. Clomipramine is effective, even in the absence of coexisting depressive symptomatology.[38][39] Trichotillomania responds to the same drug,[40] but this should not be taken as evidence that the nature of these two conditions is similar.

Tics and Tourette's syndrome

Simple motor tics are widespread, transient, and can usually be managed with explanation and reassurance. The syndrome of Gilles de la Tourette comprises multiple motor tics and phonic tics. Medication is only indicated when the tics are intrusive and handicapping. There is no evidence that early treatment modifies the course of the disease.

Haloperidol is best researched and often cited as the treatment of choice.[41] Acute extrapyramidal reactions are common and patients should be warned of the possibility of tremor, stiffness, and oculogyric crisis, all of which will respond to antiparkinsonian agents, for example procyclidine. Antiparkinsonian drugs should only be taken if these problems arise. Haloperidol can cause excessive sedation which has been termed a "fog" state.[42] Sulpiride[28] and pimozide[43] can also cause extrapyramidal reactions but are less likely to and appear to have broadly similar efficacy.[44]

Because of reports of sudden death due to arrhythmias, pimozide is less used now. Prior ECG and subsequent monitoring is advisable and a response will usually have been achieved by 8 mg in a single daily dose if it is to occur.[43]

Phonic tics are usually the first to respond to drug treatment and then complex motor tics and then simple motor tics.

Tourette's syndrome may be associated with other psychopathology, particularly obsessive compulsive symptoms. Rhythmic complex movements that appear compulsive, for example, repetitive kissing or lining up are called complex tics in the American literature, but as they seem to lie between Tourette's syndrome and obsessive compulsive disorder, they are perhaps best referred to as complex movements. Sometimes these movements are the main problem. Neuroleptics usually leave them untouched but they will often respond to clomipramine where specific treatment is required.

Tics wax and wane but some children go into "status tic", a sequence of unrelenting tics and complex movements that leaves them sore and exhausted. In the absence of a more specific remedy, chloral induced sleep will sometimes bring relief.

Clonidine has its advocates and has the advantage that it is not a neuroleptic, but there are doubts about its efficacy[45] and in my hands it causes depression and does not affect the tics at all.

Naturally there are concerns about the lifetime risk of tardive dyskinesia in this new cohort of children receiving long term neuroleptics. Drug free days once or twice a week, perhaps at weekends, are advised to diminish the lifetime weight of drug consumed. Treatment alternatives under investigation include buspirone and calcium channel blockers.

Anxiety, panic attacks, and school refusal

Situational anxieties or phobias are best treated with behavioural methods. In school refusal in the younger child, anxieties are multifactorial and early return to school is the cornerstone of management. Anxiolytics have been used but results conflict as to their efficacy. Benzodiazepines are best avoided because of their addictive potential and propensity to behavioural side effects.

Free floating anxiety and panic attacks may be associated with hyperventilation which can be assessed in the clinic. Propranolol may be helpful but is contraindicated when there is a history of asthma or arrhythmia. It has the advantage that it can be taken "as required". The tricyclic drugs, amitriptyline and imipramine can be given for their anxiolytic effects. The present generation of monoamine oxidise inhibitors (MAOIs) is difficult to use because of the food restrictions required to avoid a pressor reaction. The newer reversible inhibitors of monoamine oxidase, moclobemide for example, may render this category of drugs more available to teenage patients.

Hysterical disorders and eating disorders

Hysterical and somatising disorders are included here because they are sometimes complicated by depression, which should be diagnosed and treated in the usual way. Likewise, the depression sometimes found in chronic fatigue syndromes and anorexia nervosa. Abreaction with intravenous amylobarbitone[46] can be helpful in the management of psychogenic stupor, as it is difficult to gain therapeutic access to a patient who can neither move nor talk.[47]

There is no specific drug treatment for anorexia nervosa, but both imipramine and fluoxetine have found support in the treatment of bulimia nervosa.[48]

Elimination

The management of encopresis is not usually undertaken before age 4 years for developmental reasons. Constipation is frequently associated and laxatives may be required. The choice of laxative is important, but "sister's favourite" is often prescribed by default. The topic has been reviewed recently by Graham Clayden and is not discussed further in this chapter.[49]

Likewise, developmental considerations determine that nocturnal enuresis is not usually treated actively before age 5 years. There is abundant evidence that behavioural methods are the treatment of choice after physical causes have been rejected. Some children respond to simple star charts rewarding dry nights.

Other children require a night trainer alarm that uses the same principle as the bell and pad and is equally effective but more convenient.[50] Many districts now have enuresis clinics to provide this service. Despite the above, amitriptyline and imipramine are still widely prescribed for nocturnal enuresis by general practitioners[1] and child psychiatrists.[2] Although effective in the short term, relapse is frequent when the drug is stopped and the risk of overdose by patient or siblings is well known.[34]

There may be a place for prescribing one of these drugs in the short term—for example, to allow a child to go on a school holiday—and the same can also be said for intranasal desmopressin,[51] but with the availability of safer more effective behavioural methods the widespread use of drugs to treat nocturnal enuresis cannot be endorsed.

In daytime wetting, behavioural methods including regular potting are the mainstay of treatment, but urodynamic review should be considered, particularly when there is associated urgency. Most of the drugs used by urodynamicists can provoke nightmares.

Hyperactivity

Children with pervasive short attention span and restless, overactive, distractable behaviour meet criteria for hyperkinetic disorder according to the *International Classification of Diseases*, 9th revision[52] and attention deficit disorder in the American system *Diagnostic and Statistical Manual of Mental Disorders*, 3rd edition revised.[53] Attention deficit disorder defines a much broader group as it also includes situational expression of these problems and it is not further discussed here.

Hyperkinetic disorder, narrowly defined, is of early onset and occurred at a rate of 17 per 1000 boys aged 6–8 years in the east London study.[54] British child psychiatrists are reluctant to make this diagnosis but usually identify the conduct disorder with which it is often associated.[55] Hyperkinetic syndrome is a handicapping condition. Management is difficult and requires attention to structure and consistency which usually involves environmental manipulation. Stimulant drugs are widely used in America and, though scarcely used in Britain, are probably the best researched psychotropic drugs in use in childhood. Even if these drugs are reserved for the most severely afflicted children who show this behaviour at home, at school, and in the doctor's office, every health district has candidate patients.

After diagnosis, baseline parent and teacher ratings using the Rutter[56] or Conners scales[57] are completed, which takes a few minutes. These can be repeated serially to assess change. Methylphenidate[58] and dexamphetamine are both effective. A Yes–No effect is sought. When there is benefit it is clear, and the school dinner lady will notice if a tablet is omitted. What is more, the child's improved behaviour is likely to have a positive effect on family interaction.[59]

Methylphenidate is only available in the United Kingdom on a

95

named patient basis from the manufacturer (CIBA Laboratories, Horsham, West Sussex RH12 4AB). It has a short life and it is given in divided doses in the range 0·3–1·5 mg/kg/day starting with about 5 mg a day depending on the size of the child.[5] Appetite suppression is sometimes a problem so I usually give it after breakfast, after lunch, and maybe after school. Evening doses cause insomnia.

Reversible growth failure is reported and is probably related to high dose regimens. Nevertheless, height, weight, and blood pressure should be measured at each clinic attendance and this means the clinic should be equipped to do this. Drug holidays are recommended for one or two days at weekends if this can be tolerated and for longer periods at least once a year. Some children become tearful or depressed and others may develop obsessive compulsive behaviour or tics. Tics are usually cited as a contra-indication.[6]

Dexamphetamine is longer acting and may be given twice a day. The dose range is similar and so are the side effects. Some children tolerate one of these drugs more readily than the other. It is said that stimulants are ineffective in hyperactive children who are mentally handicapped, but a trial is still worthwhile in selected cases.[60] Although both dexamphetamine and methylphenidate are controlled drugs, dependence is not a problem with the doses described here. Low dose imipramine, 25–50 mg a day is a useful but less potent alternative.[61]

Behaviour problems in children with epilepsy

Children with epilepsy are at much greater risk of behaviour problems. The reasons for this are multiple but only drug issues are considered here.

It is profitable to review the anticonvulsants the child is taking. The behavioural side effects of carbamazepine are often associated with peak serum concentrations, and a switch to the sustained release preparation at the same total daily dose is easy to do, will seldom result in decreased seizure control[62] or deteriorating behaviour, but sometimes produces a gratifying behavioural improvement.

The behavioural side effects of phenobarbitone are well known and paediatricians hardly use it, but some adult specialists who also treat children are unfamiliar with this side effect.

Clonazepam and clobazam can both cause profound and chronic

behavioural deterioration, even pseudodementia, if parents do not decide to stop giving them. There is sometimes cross reactivity between the two compounds but sometimes not, so it is worthwhile to try a switch. Hyperactive children with learning difficulties and intractable seizures, who have been taking a benzodiazepine from an early age, are particularly at risk that the drug induced behaviour will be assumed to be constitutional.[63]

Vigabatrin has made a notable contribution to childhood psychopathology and can produce a range of problems including psychosis.

One is reluctant to treat anticonvulsant induced hyperactivity with stimulants. Dexamphetamine raises the seizure threshold and is recommended rather than methylphenidate, which is said to lower it, in the treatment of constitutionally hyperactive children with epilepsy. In practice, methylphenidate may ameliorate or alter the seizure pattern in addition to its expected effect.

Behaviour problems in children who are mentally handicapped[7]

Mentally handicapped children who present with behaviour problems can be divided conveniently into two groups; those who are being treated with drugs and those who are not. Those who are receiving drugs are probably being given too many and sometimes show the fluctuating symptoms of a subacute confusional state. Treatment comprises drug rationalisation and reduction in the shadow of tardive dyskinesia.

Children and teenagers who present with behaviour problems severe enough to warrant consideration of drug treatment will usually have self injurious behaviour or challenging behaviour if they do not have a more conventional diagnosis, for example, depression or bipolar disorder,[64] which should be treated appropriately. Sometimes there will be a more straightforward explanation, for example, toothache or departure of a familiar member of staff from a children's home.

Self injurious behaviour, such as head-banging or eye gouging, is very difficult to treat.[65] Naltrexone has been tried in recent years with some success.[4 66] Carbamazepine can also be used.[67]

Challenging behaviour usually refers to explosive and aggressive behaviour in teenagers with limited language and limited responsiveness to social cues. Management is expensive, person intensive, and requires structure, continuity, and environmental manipulation. Regular exercise may also be of help.[68] Drugs may have a role but should always be assessed with a serial record of the frequency of the target behaviours compared with a baseline taken before the drug was started.

Neuroleptics should be avoided as far as possible because of the risk of tardive dyskinesia that can follow even a short period of neuroleptic treatment at low dose. Their short term efficacy is seductive. Depending on the assessment of the problem, separate exhibition of carbamazepine,[69 70] propranolol,[71] or lithium[6 72] may all be considered.

This world of chronic handicap is swept by enthusiasms. Fenfluramine has fallen out of favour for autism,[73] but amantadine and calcium channel blockers are on the horizon.[74]

Conclusion

It is always a serious decision to recommend parents give drugs to their children. Sometimes it is a serious omission not to recommend parents give drugs to their children.

I am grateful to Mary Eminson for advice and support and to Claire Brittain for typing the manuscript.

1 Adams S. Prescribing of psychotropic drugs to children and adolescents. *BMJ* 1991;**302**:217.
2 Bramble DJ. The use of anti-depressants by British child psychiatrists. *Psychiatric Bulletin* 1992;**16**:396–8.
3 Graham P. *Child psychiatry: a developmental approach*. 2nd Ed. Oxford: Oxford University Press, 1991.
4 Gadow KD. Paediatric psychopharmacotherapy. A review of recent research. *J Child Psychol Psychiatry* 1992;**33**:153–95.
5 Hyman SE, Arana GW. *Handbook of psychiatric drug therapy*. 2nd Ed. Boston: Little Brown, 1991.
6 Green WH. *Child and adolescent clinical psychopharmacology*. Baltimore: Williams and Wilkins, 1991.
7 Gualtieri CT. *Neuropsychiatry and behavioural pharmacology*. New York: Springer-Verlag, 1991.
8 Cooper JR, Bloom FE, Roth RH. *The biochemical basis of neurophamarcology*. New York: Oxford University Press, 1991.
9 Douglas J, Richman N. *My child won't sleep*. Harmondsworth: Penguin, 1984.
10 British Medical Association and the Royal Pharmaceutical Society of Great Britain. *British national formulary*. Number 23. London: BMA and the Royal Pharmaceutical Society of Great Britain, 1992.
11 Simonoff EA, Stores G. Controlled trial of trimeprazine tartrate for night waking. *Arch Dis Child* 1987;**62**:253–7.
12 Parkes JD. *Sleep and its disorders*. London: W B Saunders, 1985:133.
13 Lask B. Novel and non-toxic treatment for night terrors. *BMJ* 1988;**297**:592.
14 Pesikoff RB, Davis PC. Treatment of pavor nocturnus and somnambulism in children. *Am J Psychiatry* 1971;**128**:778–81.

15 Puente RM. The use of carbamazepine in the treatment of behavioural disorders in children. In: Birkmayer W, ed. *Epileptic seizures, behaviour, pain.* Bern: Hans Huber Publishers 1976:243–52.

16 Alvarez B, Dahlitz M, Grimshaw J, Parkes JD. Mazindol in the long term treatment of narcolepsy. *Lancet* 1991;337:1293–4.

17 Mouret J, Sanchez P, Taillard J, Lemoine P, Robelin N, Canini F. Treatment of narcolepsy with L-tyrosine. *Lancet* 1988;ii:1458–9.

18 Elwes RDC, Chesterman LP, Jenner P, et al. Treatment of narcolepsy with L-tyrosine: double-blind placebo controlled trial. *Lancet* 1989;ii:1067–9.

19 Nelson HE, Trasher S, Barnes TRE. Practical ways of alleviating auditory hallucinations. *BMJ* 1991;302:327.

20 Garralda MI. Hallucinations in children with conduct and emotional disorders: 1. the clinical phenomena. *Psychol Med* 1984;14:589–96.

21 Garralda ME. Hallucinations in children with conduct and emotional disorders: 2. the follow-up study. *Psychol Med* 1984;14:597–604.

22 Eggers C, Ropke B. Pharmacotherapy of schizophrenia in childhood and adolescence. In: Eggers C, ed. *Schizophrenia and youth. Etiology and therapeutic consequences.* Berlin: Springer-Verlag, 1991:182–95.

23 Siefen G, Remschmidt H. Results of treatment with clozapine in schizophrenic adolescents. *Z Kinder Jugendpsychiatr* 1986;14:245–57.

24 Ciompi L. Affect logic and schizophrenia. In: Eggers C, ed. *Schizophrenia and youth. Etiology and therapeutic consequences.* Berlin: Springer-Verlag, 1991:20.

25 Kutcher SP, MacKenzie S, Galarraga W, Szalai J. Clonazepam treatment of adolescents with neuroleptic induced akathisia. *Am J Psychiatry* 1987;144:823–4.

26 Turk J, Lask B. Neuroleptic malignant syndrome. *Arch Dis Child* 1991;66:91–2.

27 Perry R, Campbell M, Green WH, et al. Neuroleptic related dyskinesias in autistic children: a prospective study. *Psychopharmacol Bull* 1985;21:140–3.

28 Lees AJ. *Tics and related disorders.* Edinburgh: Churchill Livingstone, 1985.

29 Carlson GA. Child and adolescent mania—diagnostic considerations. *J Child Psychol Psychiatry* 1990;31:331–41.

30 Varanka TM, Weller RA, Weller EB, Fristad MA. Lithium treatment of manic episodes with psychotic features in pre-pubertal children. *Am J Psychiatry* 1988;145:1557–9.

31 Srinivasan DP, Abaya V, Birch NJ. Lithium therapy update. *Hospital Update* 1992;18:300–4.

32 Crawford R, Silverstone T. Carbamazepine in affective disorder. *International Journal of Clinical Psychopharmacology* 1987;2(suppl 1).

32a Pope HG, McElroy SL, Keck PE, Hudson JI. Valproate in the treatment of acute mania. A placebo controlled study. *Arch Gen Psychiatry* 1991;48:62–80.

32b Harrington RC. The natural history and treatment of child and adolescent affective disorders. *J Child Psychol Psychiatry* 1992;33:1287–302.

33 Puig-Antich J, Perel JM, Lupatkin W, et al. Imipramine in pre-pubertal major depressive disorders. *Arch Gen Psychiatry* 1987;44:81–9.

34 Giles H McC. Imipramine poisoning in childhood. *BMJ* 1963;ii:844–6.

35 Leibenluft B, Wehr TA. Is sleep deprivation useful in the treatment of depression? *Am J Psychiatry* 1992;149:159–68.

36 King BH, Baxter LR, Stuber M, Fish B. Therapeutic sleep deprivation for depression in children. *J Am Acad Child Adolesc Psychiatry* 1987;26:928–31.

37 Bertagnoli MW, Borchardt CM. A review of ECT for children and adolescents. *J Am Acad Child Adolesc Psychiatry* 1990;29:302–7.

38 Flament MF, Rapoport JL, Berg CJ, et al. Clomipramine treatment of childhood obsessive compulsive disorder. *Arch Gen Psychiatry* 1985;42:977–83.

39 DeVeaugh-Geiss J, Moroz G, Biederman J, et al. Clomipramine hydrochloride

in childhood and adolescent obsessive compulsive disorder—a multicentre trial. *J Am Acad Child Adolesc Psychiatry* 1992;**31**:45–9.

40 Swedo SE, Rapoport JL. Trichotillomania. *J Child Psychol Psychiatry* 1991;**32**:401–9.

41 Shapiro AK, Shapiro E. Treatment of tic disorders with haloperidol. In: Cohen DJ, Bruun RD, Leckmann JF, eds. *Tourette's syndrome and tic disorders: clinical understanding and treatment.* New York: J Wiley, 1988:268–80.

42 Bruun RD. Subtle and underrecognised side effects of neuroleptic treatment in children with Tourette's disorder. *Am J Psychiatry* 1988;**145**:621–4.

43 Moldofsky H, Sandor P. Pimozide in the treatment of Tourette's syndrome. In: Cohen DJ, Bruun RD, Leckman JF, eds. *Tourette's syndrome and tic disorders: clinical understanding and treatment.* New York: J Wiley, 1988:282–9.

44 Shapiro E, Shapiro AK, Fulop G, et al. Controlled study of haloperidol, pimozide and placebo for the treatment of Gilles de la Tourette syndrome. *Arch Gen Psychiatry* 1989;**46**:722–30.

45 Leckman JF, Walkup JT, Cohen DJ. Clonidine treatment of Tourette's syndrome. In: Cohen DJ, Bruun RD, Leckman JF, eds. *Tourette's syndrome and tic disorders: clinical understanding and treatment.* New York: J Wiley, 1988:292–301.

46 Perry C, Jacobs D. Overview: clinical applications of the amytal interview in psychiatric emergency settings. *Am J Psychiatry* 1982;**139**:552–9.

47 White A, Corbin DOC, Coope B. The use of thiopentone in the treatment of non-organic locomotor disorders. *J Psychosom Res* 1988;**32**:249–53.

48 Goldbloom DS, Kennedy SH, Kaplan AS, Woodside DB. Anorexia nervosa and bulimia nervosa. *Can Med Assoc J* 1989;**140**:1149–54.

49 Clayden GS. Management of chronic constipation. *Arch Dis Child* 1992;**67**:340–4.

50 Fordham KE, Meadow SR. Controlled study of standard pad and bell alarm against mini alarm for nocturnal enuresis. *Arch Dis Child* 1989;**64**:651–6.

51 Evans JHC, Meadow SR. Desmopressin for bed wetting: length of treatment, vasopressin secretion, and response. *Arch Dis Child* 1992;**67**:184–8.

52 World Health Organisation. *Mental disorders: glossary and guide to the classification in accordance with the ninth revision of the international classification of diseases.* Geneva: WHO, 1978.

53 American Psychiatric Association. *Diagnostic and statistical manual of mental disorders (DSM-III-R).* 3rd Ed, revised. Washington DC: American Psychiatric Association 1987.

54 Taylor E, Sandberg S, Thorley G, Giles S. *The epidemiology of childhood hyperactivity.* Institute of Psychiatry Maudsley Monographs. London: Oxford University Press, 1991.

55 Prendergast M, Taylor E, Rapoport JL, et al. The diagnosis of childhood hyperactivity: a US–UK cross national study of DSM-III and ICD-9. *J Child Psychol Psychiatry* 1988;**29**:289–300.

56 Rutter M, Tizard J, Whitmore K, eds. *Education, health and behaviour.* London: Longmans Green, 1970.

57 Goyette CH, Conners CK, Ulrich RF. Normative data on revised parent and teacher rating scales. *J Abnorm Child Psychol* 1978;**6**:221–36.

58 Taylor E, Schachar R, Thorley G, Wieselberg HM, Everitt B, Rutter M. Which boys respond to stimulant medication? A controlled trial of methylphenidate in boys with disruptive behaviour. *Psychol Med* 1987;**17**:121–43.

59 Schachar R, Taylor E, Wieselberg M, Thorley G, Rutter M. Changes in family function and relationships in children who respond to methylphenidate. *J Am Acad Child Adolesc Psychiatry* 1987;**26**:728–32.

60 Gadow KD, Poling E. *Pharamcotherapy and mental retardation.* Boston: College Hill Press, 1988.

61 Rapoport JL, Quinn PO, Bradbard G, Riddle D, Brookes E. Imipramine and methylphenidate treatments of hyperactive boys: a double-blind comparison. *Arch Gen Psychiatry* 1974;**30**:789–93.

62 Ryan SW, Forsythe I, Hartley R, Haworth M, Bowmer CJ. Slow release carbamazepine in treatment of poorly controlled seizures. *Arch Dis Child* 1990;**65**:930–5.

63 Commander M, Green SH, Prendergast M. Behavioural disturbances in children treated with clonazepam. *Dev Med Child Neurol* 1991;**33**:362–3.

64 McCracken JT, Diamond RP. Bipolar disorder in mentally retarded adolescents. *J Am Acad Child Adolesc Psychiatry* 1988;**27**:494–9.

65 Farber JM. Psychopharmacology of self injurious behaviour in the mentally retarded. *J Am Acad Child Adolesc Psychiatry* 1987;**26**:296–302.

66 Barrett RP, Feinstein C, Hole WT. Effects of naloxone and naltrexone on self injury: a double blind placebo controlled analysis. *Am J Ment Retard* 1989;**93**:644–51.

67 Barrett RP, Payton JB, Burkhart JE: Treatment of self injury and disruptive behaviour with carbamazepine (Tegretol) and behaviour therapy. *Journal of the Multi-handicapped Person* 1988;**1**:79–91.

68 McGimsey JF, Favell JE. The effects of increased physical exercise on disruptive behaviour in retarded persons. *J Autism Dev Disord* 1988;**18**:167–79.

69 Evans RW, Clay TH, Gualtieri CT. Carbamazepine in pediatric psychiatry. *J Am Acad Child Adolesc Psychiatry* 1987;**26**:2–8.

70 Sovner R. Use of anticonvulsant agents for the treatment of neuropsychiatric disorders in the developmentally disabled. In: Ratey JJ, ed. *Mental retardation: developing phamacotherapies*. Washington DC: American Psychiatric Press, 1991:83–106.

71 Ratey JJ, Lindem KJ. Beta blockers as primary treatment for aggression and self injury in the developmentally disabled. In: Ratey JJ, ed. *Mental retardation: developing pharmacotherapies*. Washington DC: American Psychiatric Press, 1991:51–81.

72 Tyrer SP, Walsh A, Edwards DE, Berney TP, Stephens DA. Factors associated with a good response to lithium in aggressive mentally handicapped subjects. *Progress in Neuropsychopharmacology* 1984;**8**:751–5.

73 Aman MG, Kern RA. Review of fenfluramine in the treatment of developmental disabilities. *J Am Acad Child Psychiatry* 1989;**28**:549–65.

74 Chandler M, Barnhill LJ, Gaultieri CT. Amantadine: profile of use in the developmentally disabled. In: Ratey JJ, ed. *Mental retardation developing pharmacotherapies*. Washington DC: American Psychiatric Press, 1991:139–62.

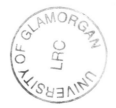

8. Inpatient treatment: personal practice

Jonathan Green

Introduction

Inpatient child psychiatry should be seen as a specific mode of treatment in its own right, rather than a convenient way of delivering other treatments, or a form of substitute care. The kind of therapeutic work and research generated within inpatient units has taken a distinguished place in the history of mental health services for children,[1] but in the current climate there are several trends that quite rightly require those of us working in such units to clarify and define our role in current mental health services for children. In both paediatrics and adult mental health there has been a move away from inpatient beds and towards primary care and community services. In child psychiatry the usual family oriented approach can make isolating the child during an admission seem paradoxical. Our units, although low on medical technology, have high needs for staffing and physical fabric, and can seem expensive.

As in any mode of treatment, we can conveniently consider indications for use, mode of action, appropriate "dosage", efficacy, and unwanted effects. The focus of this chapter is child inpatient units taking children up to 14 years old; adolescent psychiatry units taking children from 14 upwards have their own particular features, although many of the same points apply.

Indications for inpatient treatment

In practice, the decision to admit a patient to a unit balances the anxieties of referrer and family about the intolerability or dangerousness of a psychological state against the appropriateness of admission as a solution and the unit's capacity to take over the patient's care.

> ## Box 1—Indications for inpatient treatment
>
> Severe persistent life-threatening disorders (depression/suicide, eating disorders, obsessional disorders, intractible soiling, psychotic illness, hysterical conversion)
>
> Clarification of diagnosis or treatment indications (severe emotional disorders with complex family pathology, autistic-like and other neuropsychiatric disorders, assessment of parenting where there is risk for the child as in Munchausen's syndrome by proxy)
>
> Crisis situations
>
> Controlled trials of drug treatments.

Most admissions will fall into one of these groups:

(1) Problems for which outpatient treatment is felt to be insufficient or impossible and where there is a need for the intensity, wide range, or safety of residential therapy involving nursing staff. The child's disorder is sometimes life threatening, usually severe or persistent: such as serious depression or suicidal risk, eating disorder, obsessional disorders, intractable soiling, psychotic illness, or hysterical conversion.

(2) Problems where the nature of the difficulties is not clear and residential assessment could be a valuable aid in clarifying the diagnosis and the treatment needed. Examples here would be some severe emotional disorders with complex family pathology; autistic-like syndromes; neuropsychiatric disorders where the balance between organic and psychological factors is not clear; and the assessment of parenting, using the whole team in structured assessments that are described below.

(3) Crisis situations in which psychological disorder in the child or family has reached such a pitch that caring has broken down, the child is at risk, and the referrer highly concerned. This is using the unit as "asylum". An important distinction has to be made here between family breakdown in the context of psychiatric treatment, and care and control issues where reception into social services care would be more appropriate.

(4) Occasional admission for controlled trials of drug treatment such as stimulants or for supervised alteration of antipsychotic or anticonvulsant medication.

Despite calls from within the profession for more consistency,[23] inpatient units have often tended to develop idiosyncratically according to local conditions and personalities. Most units will develop a preferred way of working and an expertise, which will

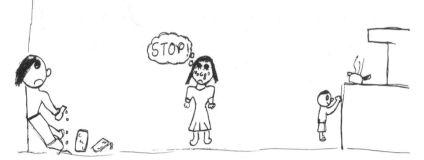

"Mum's been drinking." Children may become deeply despondent about responsibilities put on them by a major breakdown in parenting

generate biases in referral and patient selection. I think that it is crucial for the legitimacy of these scarce (usually supradistrict) resources, however, that they maintain the flexibility to respond to a full range of referrer need.

How are inpatient units therapeutic?

A family orientation

In the past, many psychiatric units created communities which were an "alternative world" for the child during the course of long admissions over several years. The intention was for children to experience alternative care and a specialised social life that would allow them to recover from a traumatic external environment. Such environments can be valuable and still exist,[4] but on the whole not within the health service. Current inpatient units usually see themselves as providing shorter admissions, and as being more flexibly integrated with the child's usual environment and local service provision.[5] This is particularly the case in relation to the family. Inpatient units face two ways: inwards towards providing a specialised therapeutic environment for the child, but also outwards towards working with the family and preparing them from the outset for the child's return. This Janus faced position is arduous but essential to maintain. The paradox of the child leaving home temporarily the better to return, influences our whole practice, and the implications of working with parents under the Children Act 1989 have only strengthened this orientation. The Act emphasises the continuing central role of parents when children are away from home and the need for services to work in partnership with families at all times.[6]

A child will thus only be admitted to the unit when there is an effective home base with which to work and to where the child can be discharged (this may need to be a social services provision if the family has completely broken down).

The therapeutic effect of separation

Temporary separation of child from family is clearly one of the identifying features of inpatient, as compared to other, treatments. Children become resident for substantial lengths of time (mean length of admission in my unit is about nine weeks but many treatments will extend for five months or more). This time away from family and school can have profoundly useful consequences. The children have a chance to experience themselves in a therapeutic environment. The family has a chance to recover and change without the continual pressure of crises. If effective work has been accomplished with both child and family, then the way is potentially open for a more positive reintegration of the child into the family by the end of treatment.

The admission process

We attempt to maximise the therapeutic potential of this separation, and minimise any potential harmful effects, by undertaking considerable work in assessing the family before the admission and negotiating with them and the referrer about it. Problems are clarified, general aims are set, and the responsibilities of other family members to work with the unit during admission are defined. Sometimes a formal "contract" is produced and signed. As Bruggen et al have described,[7 8] this preadmission work can be very effective at focusing minds and sometimes obviates the necessity for admission at all. This is worth stressing because referrers to inpatient units (as well as families) often expect an immediate admission rather along the model of the medical ward and may feel frustrated by what are seen as obstructive preadmission procedures.

A conventional emergency admission service is nevertheless available, and children can be assessed and admitted within a few hours when necessary. (Usually the urgency relates to the safety of the child or others.) After such an admission the usual preadmission procedure will still be undertaken before a further commitment is made to keep the child for longer therapy.

Therapeutic milieu: the unit as "parent"

Theoretical writing on inpatient units has tended to oscillate between seeing the ward environment as a neutral background to specific treatments,[5] or as the major therapeutic agent in itself. Wards have been developed to function therapeutically in two major ways. In the therapeutic community model, derived from pioneering work after the war in adult psychiatry, the living among other patients and staff itself, when properly supervised and explored in groups, is seen to have a major role in social learning and psychological readjustment.[9] In a ward run on behaviour modification lines, however, the contingencies on particular behaviours are carefully controlled so as to produce specific change in that behaviour.

I do not think that the therapeutic community approach, in its extreme form, is appropriate for young and disturbed children whose major lack has often been good parenting. On the other hand the behaviour modification model, while useful symptomatically, does not address the deeper emotional needs of many of our children. I prefer to think of the unit acting as "parent"; a role that goes beyond the inevitable sense of a residential unit being "in loco parentis" to a psychological orientation that has implications for the nursing approach, staff organisation and communication, and the physical environment of the ward.

Parenting is a complex series of skills. Most parents use at various times short range tactics aimed at rapidly modifying behaviour (the promise of a treat, a raised voice); medium range strategies involving organisation in space and time for children and communicating clear expectations; and long range goals, at the deepest level, to foster attachments and relationships. I see the unit doing likewise. We use behavioural methods in a planned way to modify specific behaviours. We recognise that the organisation and purposefulness of the environment can reduce unnecessary aggression and promote positive group dynamics. We then make space for privacy and individual nurturing that responds to the children's need for attachment and intimacy, recognising that this is often the deepest level at which they have suffered. The importance of peer relationships can be fostered by means of community groups and joint projects. Within such an environment, we find no need for a "time out" room, in the behaviour modification sense; we use a supervised quiet room for children to "cool down" when group tensions become explosive.

Staff need to show the kind of adult behaviour that research suggests promotes effective parenting; consistency of approach, good communication between the adults, clear communication of expectations and boundaries to the children, firmness without retaliation or aggression, and the provision of appropriate privacy and time for intimate nurturing and physical care.

A very high quality of work and organisation is required to preserve this kind of "parental stance" in the face of assaults, retaliation, acting out, despair, and provocation from the children individually or, more powerfully, as a group. The children are organised into age orientated groups who have their own space on the unit and are worked with by a specific staff team. There is maximum autonomy and devolved responsibility within that staff team: this is because the treatment is delivered essentially through individual relationships between adult and child, and these relationships are only possible for staff if they have a sense of personal responsibility for their actions within shared treatment aims.[10] Leadership and supervision are needed from senior staff at all times.

The physical environment is also important. Many psychiatric wards are often shabby and hidden away "around the back". Management must be recruited effectively to counter this as the physical environment is a vital part of the treatment; an environment that is cared for sends a subliminal message of care to the children within it.[11] Bettleheim famously used the best cutlery and furnishings in his orthogenic school (even though they might not last long!) for just this reason.[12]

The discharge phase

The relationship between child, family, and ward typically will have gone through a number of stages during the admission. Initially the parents may be relieved, and the child and the ward will be accommodating to each other. In the intense treatment phase the child can sometimes become strongly attached to the ward and active work with the family is needed at this stage to prevent splits and to maintain morale: a specific group for parents is also very helpful. Towards discharge there will be a reintegration phase, when the child prepares to leave the ward (which has often come to feel safe) and parents take back increasing responsibility again. The ward will offer a follow up phase of continuing contact, home visiting, and school liaison as necessary. For a minority of children, full integration back home is not practicable and the admission proves to be a stepping stone to long term residential placement or other care.

Specific therapeutic programmes

In addition to this general milieu and family work, the inpatient unit offers a range of other specific treatments. These will include individual child psychotherapy, behavioural programmes, medication, group work and creative work on the wards, work between parent and child, family therapy, and specific parent groups[13] (see other chapters in this book). All children are medically assessed and investigated where necessary. The unit's school is specifically for children on the ward and provides educational assessment and teaching, in liaison with the child's own school.

To coordinate these different specific treatments an important topic of current developments in many units is "focal treatment planning".[14-16] Goals are carefully defined before admission, treatments designed to accomplish these goals, and progress reviewed. This planning aims to avoid interminable treatment and therapeutic "drift" by setting out achievable and measurable aims. In our unit at Booth Hall hospital, much work focuses around several assessment and therapy programmes—for instance, a parenting programme, a programme for autistic-like social impairments, and a programme for overactivity disorders. These programmes organise the staff into specific patterns of assessment and care and, because of their uniformity, make research into the delivery and outcome of treatment much easier. They also present a clear service to referrers that can be costed. For children whose needs fall outside these programmes, the care plan will be individualised; but the goal orientation and monitoring is the same.

The parenting programme illustrates how the resources of an inpatient unit can be used in this kind of structured package. During the assessment (a) the parents are seen individually as outpatients; (b) children's developmental and psychological states are assessed by ward and teaching staff, usually during a sequence of daypatient stays; and (c) a brief residential admission of the whole family is used to make direct nursing observations of parenting and family interactions in a structured setting, observations that compliment home based observations made previously. These separate assessments are then integrated to provide an overall formulation of difficulties, which guides the feedback to the family and any treatment planning. The treatment itself may use group, individual, or family methods, as indicated by the assess-

> ## Box 2—Treatment strategies in inpatient units
>
> Maintaining family involvement: —preadmission negotiation
> —family therapy
> —parents groups
>
> Milieu treatment: the unit as a parent
> - Consistency of approach
> - Good communication between adults
> - Clear communication of expectations and boundaries
> - Firmness without retaliation or aggression
> - Provision of appropriate privacy
> - Time for intimate nurturing and physical care.
>
> Specific treatment strategies:
> - structured packages of assessment and care
> - individual child therapy
> - group therapy
> - behavioural programmes
> - medication.

ment. Commonly, intensive parent training or relationship work will be undertaken by ward staff during day attendance of parents alongside the child, and in parallel with individual therapy. In some cases a further formal assessment period will be undertaken at the end of treatment, to judge progress.

Unwanted effects of inpatient treatment

Like any powerful therapy, inpatient treatment can have unwanted effects. It may prescribed in the wrong situation, and this is usually the result of inadequate preadmission assessment. The admission of a child, for instance, may simply collude with a scapegoating rejection by the family. Removal of a child from a local school for admission may take away the only source of real continuity and esteem that he or she has. The treatment may be continued too long and child and family may become demoralised or the child resigned to the institution or the sick role.

The dynamics of a unit can become unhelpful in several ways. Especially working with deprived groups, there is a tendency to become introverted and self contained, preoccupied with "rescuing" children from an environment that is increasingly seen to be harsh and uncaring. Attitudes can drift into "parent blaming" (PS Penfold, presentation to 9th Congress of the European Society for Child and Adolescent Psychiatry, London 1991), longer admissions, and anxious overprotection of the children; in effect a substitute care. We work against this tendency by the involvement of ward staff in community visiting and home visits, and the active engagement of families into treatment alongside the child. Of course, the reality *is* often appalling. We have to recognise the powerful feelings that these children evoke in us, the pain their predicament can provoke, and, most of all, the limitations of what we can sometimes do. A well functioning team can be very helpful here: listening to each other's distress and clarifying issues. A team functioning poorly will often not recognise that it is mirroring the child or family psychopathology in its own process, and the despair is compounded. Main's classic paper describes this well.[17]

A second, related, way in which the treatment can go wrong is in the therapeutic drift that comes from unclear goals or a difficulty in appropriately placing children who cannot return to their families, at a time when social services resources are diminishing.

Thirdly, the "parental care" of the unit can fail under stress: demoralisation and disintegration of care set in, the emphasis switch from care and treatment to custodial control, and the fabric of the unit deteriorate. Here the stage is set for the excesses of institutional abuse which have been at times associated with residential environments. Prevention lies in leadership, a clear unit ethos, supervision and support from experienced staff, and in good staff recruitment.

Finally, inpatient units can sometimes be denigrated along with their patients, seen as places of "last resort", and become overloaded with "impossible" intractable problems. This obviously promotes demoralisation. The answer lies in patient selection, and a more active approach to the use of intensive treatment earlier in the course of psychopathology. The inpatient unit should not be seen as the end of the line, but rather an "intensive therapy unit" where work can be undertaken at any stage in the development of psychiatric disorder.

How effective is inpatient treatment?

Several studies have looked at the efficacy of inpatient treatment.[18-22] There are great methodological problems in patient selection, comparison treatment groups, and the measurements of outcome. There has not been a prospective randomised study of inpatient compared with community care for a particular disorder, although one is now being planned in the United Kingdom. In general, studies show beneficial treatment effects, particularly with less severe disorders, and when there is specialised treatment programming and good aftercare. In severe disorders, a good "health gain" can include the accurate identification of ongoing treatment needs. One provocative finding suggests that the length of admission has only a modest relation to outcome.[20] This kind of result has led to suggestions of standard admission lengths for all patients.[13] This is rigid, and many severely disturbed children undoubtedly benefit from longer admissions, but cost/benefit analysis of longer stays is bound to become an increasing concern.

Conclusions

The child psychiatry team has little in the way of technology to fall back on to effect cures. Medication has its place, but by and large the efficacy of our treatment relies on a psychological momentum generated and sustained within the staff group, the group of children, and their families. The power, but also sometimes the weakness, of inpatient treatment lies in the size and intensity of this group process. Like any treatment it has drawbacks, but if these are recognised and the treatment prescribed appropriately, it can work powerful change. For obvious reasons the unit is an excellent source of training and teaching (at any one time our unit is training five psychiatric social work students, one psychology student, four training psychiatrists, and several learning nurses). It is potentially an excellent environment for the development and evaluation of new treatments and for scientific research. In this latter context, it has great value as a place where children's behaviour can be observed precisely, as part of assessment and during treatment.

The future vitality of inpatient unit treatment will depend on a sensitivity to changing needs in referrers, and demonstration of the superiority, in certain disorders, of this form of assessment and treatment over alternatives. At its best, a well functioning inpatient unit can have an effect on child mental health that is considerably beyond the actual number of children in a region who pass through it. This will occur partly through research and training, but there is also an indefinable sense of the unit "being there" as a resource and support for other professionals.

It is a pleasure to acknowledge that most of the ideas and practices described here were developed in collaboration with members of the inpatient team at Booth Hall Hospital.

My thanks to Sister Maureen Burke and to Dr Michael Morton for their helpful comments on early drafts of the chapter.

1 Wardle CJ. 20th Century influences on the development in Britain of services for child and adolescent psychiatry. *Br J Psychiatry* 1991;**159**:53–68.
2 Wrate RM, Wolkind S. Child and adolescent psychiatry in-patient units. *Psychiatric Bulletin* 1991;**15**:36.
3 Health Advisory Service Report on Services for Disturbed Adolescents. *Bridges over troubled waters*. London: HMSO, 1986.
4 Rose M. 1990. *Healing hurt minds: the Peper Harow experience*. London: Tavistock/Routledge, 1990.
5 Hersov L, Bentovim A. Inpatient and day-hospital units. In: Rutter M, Hersov L, eds. *Child and adolescent psychiatry, modern approaches*, Oxford: Blackwell Scientific Publications, 1985.
6 Department of Health. *The Children Act 1991: an introductory guide*. London: HMSO, 1991.
7 Bruggen P, Byng-Hall J, Pitt-Aitkens T. The reason for admission as a focus of work for an adolescent unit. *Br J Psychiatry* 1973;**123**:319–29.
8 Bruggen P, O'Brien C. *Helping families. Systems, residential and agency responsiblity*. London: Faber, 1987.
9 Kennard D. An introduction to therapeutic communities. London: Routledge and Kegan Paul, 1983.
10 Menzies-Lyth I. *Containing anxiety in institutions: selected essays*. Vol 1. London: Free Association Books, 1979.
11 Cotton NS, Geraty RG. Therapeutic space design in an inpatient unit. *Am J Orthopsychiatry* 1984;**54**:624–36.
12 Bettleheim B. *The empty fortress*. New York: Free Press, 1973.
13 Ney PG, Mulvihill DL. *Child psychiatry treatment: a practical guide*. London: Croom Helm, 1985.
14 Harper G. Focal inpatient treatment planning. *J Am Acad Child Adolesc Psychiatry* 1989;**28**:38–47.
15 Nurcombe B. Goal directed treatment planning and the principles of brief hospitalisation. *J Am Acad Child Adolesc Psychiatry* 1989;**28**:26–30.
16 Woolston JL. Transactional risk model for short and intermediate term psychiatric inpatient treatment of children. *J Am Acad Child Adolesc Psychiatry* 1989;**28**:38–41.
17 Main TE. The ailment. *Br J Med Psychol* 1957;**30**:129–45.
18 Pfeiffer SI, Strzelecki SC. Inpatient psychiatric treatment of children and adolescents: a review of outcome studies. *J Am Acad Child Adolesc Psychiatry* 1990;**29**:847–53.
19 Pfeiffer SI. Follow up of children and adolescents treated in psychiatric facilities: a methodology review. *The Psychiatric Hospital* 1989;**20**:15–20.
20 Blotchy MJ, Dimperio TL, Gossett JT. The follow up of children treated in psychiatric hospitals: a review of studies. *Am J Psychiatry* 1984;**141**:1499–507.
21 Windsberg BG, Bialer I, Cukupietzs, Botti E, Balka EB. Home versus hospital care of children with behaviour disorders. *Arch Gen Psychiatry* 1980;**37**:413–8.
22 Kazdin AE. Hospitalisation of anti-social children: clinical cause, follow-up status, and predictors of outcome. *Behav Res Ther* 1989;**11**:1–67.

PART III

LIAISING WITH OTHER SERVICES

9. Consultative work in child and adolescent psychiatry

Derek Steinberg

It should be said at the outset in a chapter in a book on treatment that, of course, consultation is not a form of therapy. Indeed, in some important ways it can be seen as, at times, an alternative to therapy.

Because of the nature of the problems with which they deal, and because of the relatively ill defined (and perhaps undefinable) boundaries to their professional territory, psychiatrists are approached about a much wider range of problems than are attributable to psychiatric disorder, or which need psychiatric care. Every seriously unhappy or misbehaving child *could* at least in principle be taken on by a child psychiatrist. This, however, would make no more sense than to say that the "right" professional would be a psychologist, psychotherapist, family therapist, paediatrician, general practitioner, health visitor, or counsellor with the appropriate skills and interests, for that matter. (And there are some 30 or 40 other workers one could list.) It often is not clear who is in the best position to help which child and family with whatever presents as a psychiatric problem. It depends not only on the clinical symptomatology, if any, but on the skills, strengths, availability, motivation, and interests of the other people involved with the child. This includes his or her parents and non-clinicians such as teachers.

The value of consultative approaches is that they can clarify who is in the best position to deal with a given problem, and help them to do so.

The nature of consultation

In this context the term consultation represents a set of techniques and approaches by which one professional can help another,

---

Box 1—Indications for a consultative approach

- When most of the required skills are probably already there or potentially there (eg consultation with paediatrics)
- When it seems that continuity with existing care givers is likely to be more productive than offering sessional therapy (eg consultation with the staff of a children's home or school)
- When there is agreement on both sides that staff education and development around the problem in question would be welcomed (eg consultation with a child development or mental handicap team, or where any team identifies for itself a need for focused in-service training of this sort)
- Where most or all of the necessary information is already with the referring team, and a comprehensive clinical reassessment seems less important than a joint review of how best to proceed (eg consultation between child and adult psychiatric or medical services)
- When rationalisation of the use of specialist and secondary or tertiary services seems sensible.

---

not necessarily by taking over the child's case (although this can remain an option), but by seeing if he or she can help the first worker to manage the child's case after all. At the most basic descriptive level, consultation is about one professional (the consultant) helping another (the consultee) with a problem but without taking over care or professional responsibility. In this sense it differs from traditional *clinical* consultation, where the doctor sees and treats the patient. To avoid confusion I have recommended the term *interprofessional consultation*[1] for the work described here.

What is interesting about interprofessional consultation (and having thus identifed it, I will revert to "consultation" for short) is the complex range of implications of this relatively simple and straightforward definition. Consultation could involve, for example, a child psychiatrist and a paediatrician discussing a case in a way that leaves the referring professional feeling that he or she would like to carry on with the patient concerned and reasonably confident about doing so. In this example, the consultant may have helped the consultee appreciate what he or she can after all do for a child who was thought at first to need psychiatric care. But consultation can also involve a visiting doctor helping the staff of, for example, a school or children's home develop ways of handling a misbehaving boy effectively enough to avoid him having to be seen at a psychiatric clinic; and as a result, ideally, handling a proportion of other children more effectively too.

This may invite the question whether consultation is no more than a substitute for clear criteria for referral to a psychiatric clinic. However, though the criteria, say, for the referral of a child with the symptoms of meningitis or appendicitis from a generalist to a specialist are clear, decisions about when or whether people have reached the limits of their resources in handling unhappy, misbehaving, or otherwise malfunctioning children are less clear cut. The consultative process brings in a whole set of other variables, such as ideas, imagination, problem solving skills, staff consistency and, not least, opportunities (or the lack of them) to get together and consider what to do in a reasonably calm, systematic, and focused way. It is a constant surprise in consultative work to find how often staff involved in child care can do more than they initially thought, when the only authority the outside consultant brings is "permission" to stand back for half an hour from the tension and hurly-burly of the work, and the skill to help them look again at what they are trying to do and how they are trying to do it.[1-3]

This implies a further important characteristic of consultative work: that the point is not for the consultant to bring his or her own methods and concepts to bear on the issue at hand, *but to seek to mobilise those of the consultees.* The psychiatrist consulting to, say, a paediatric clinic, school, or children's home doesn't try to treat the children "through" the paediatrician, teachers, or residential staff but uses consultative approaches to mobilise paediatric, teaching, or residential care experience and skill.

Box 2—Strategies for interprofessional consultation

- Identify other agencies already involved or which could helpfully be involved
- Establish links with key professional colleagues
- Agree what needs to be on the agenda
- Achieve reciprocity between consultant and consultee, including who is able and willing to do what
- Help mobilise or re-establish consultee's skills
- Promote a problem solving, mutually educational, approach to the subject
- Facilitate referral to specialist services where needed.

Of course, at first sight this may seem like a professional ploy akin to a jobbing gardener persuading his employer to do the digging, perhaps indicating that providing a better spade for the employer and a deckchair for the gardener might not come amiss. However, a central point in consultation is that any of us may be able to manage a particular case or issue better than we initially supposed given a focused opportunity, encouragement, and help in what is essentially a problem solving exercise. If this works, and the admittedly limited research into consultation suggests that it can,[2-5] then the consultative process is an educational exercise as well as a way of handling day to day practical matters. Instead of being told what to do, shown what to do, or having the job taken over by someone who is supposedly more expert, the consultee *learns* something new. All of us, in our roles as teachers or trainees, know that this is an effective style of training, applicable to many (though not all) situations.

There is also an important reciprocity in the consultative rela-

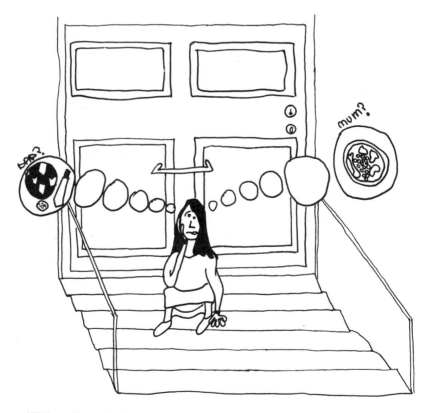

"Who to live with?" Psychiatrists may help other services attend to needs of children in disturbing situations

tionship. The person who for this particular issue is the consultant does not take a superior stance, for example indicating that the other person should surely be able to work it out for himself. Rather, the joint exploration of what a colleague has indicated is a problem is a learning exercise for the consultant too. The outcome of, say, a surgeon consulting in this way with a physician should mean that each learns something about the other's work that they didn't know before. I would say that the most important single quality of a good consultant is curiosity; a genuine wish to find out what goes on in the other's specialty, the nature of the problems that arise, how they might be clarified, and how resolved.

The value of consultation

There are benefits of consultation that—potentially—make the whole exercise worth while. I say potentially because the field is relatively new, that is about 20 years from its inception, and needs more evaluative research. But on the face of it we can suggest the following advantages:

(1) As already indicated, it can be educational. If I set out to refer an anxiety-making diabetic adolescent to a physician and, instead, the physician helped me consider how I can help the adolescent and the family manage the diabetes more effectively and responsibly, then I would learn a great deal more than had the other doctor simply taken over. I might well find that I not only handle that patient's case better, but future cases too.

(2) It may enable the patient to stay with the original practitioner instead of having another appointment with another clinician in another unit or hospital. How much time is taken up by patients in transit, or "stacked" around clinics? This is not only a question of the convenience of those involved, but also concerns continuity of care, which is of particular importance in child and adolescent psychiatry, whether we are trying to ensure stability of relationships or the success of a behaviour therapy programme. (For example autistic, unhappy, or misbehaving children are more likely to benefit from those in touch with them doing the right thing throughout the week, than from a psychiatrist doing something brilliant once a week in the clinic.)

(3) If it should emerge, immediately in consultation or later on, that the patient (or an aspect of care) would indeed be best taken over by the second professional worker, then the small amount of

119

time "lost" in consultation is likely to have been well spent in clarifying the nature of the problem, who should be doing what, and (of special importance in the child psychiatry field) who will give appropriate authority for action—for example, admission or medication. Certainly in "emergencies" in adolescent psychiatry the gains can be seen to outstrip the imagined problems when an admission to hospital, or an urgent and unplanned appointment, is held off for a little to allow for consultation between those already involved and those who are about to become involved.[6-9]

As was mentioned earlier, there are many different types of worker in the broad field of child care and mental and physical health. The field is kaleidoscopic. If the first professional approached (and this too is quite arbitrary—he or she may happen to be for example a teacher, health visitor, general practitioner, paediatrician, psychiatrist, psychologist, or counsellor, among others) feels out of his or her depth, it is often not absolutely clear to whom a new referral should be made. If the art of good consultation were part of the professional repertoire of all such specialist workers, it might well be possible to make more economical and more speedy use of the immensely complex network of different types of skill and service that we have.

(4) There is another value of consultation which I will refer to only briefly. So far I have suggested consultation as an effective way of problem solving and establishing the most appropriate help available. However, there is a great deal of ethical as well as technical controversy in medicine, and dilemmas—for example, about behaviour, education, social and family norms and expectations, HIV testing, genetic issues, high technology health care, alternative medicine, and sexual experience and behaviour—that cannot be resolved by negotiation and information alone. The subjective views and the values of different practitioners, families, and indeed children themselves also need taking into account, and again the consultative process provides a forum for sorting out not only what is supposedly needed but what is wanted. Questions of the law relating to children[10] and of informed consent[11] can also be addressed in this way.

To sum up what is being presented as the value of consultation: in an increasingly complex, diverse, and changing pattern of need on the one hand and services on the other, consultation can be a more effective way than the traditional "referral" of sorting out who is most able and willing to do what. And, further, it is a method that educates all sides as it proceeds.

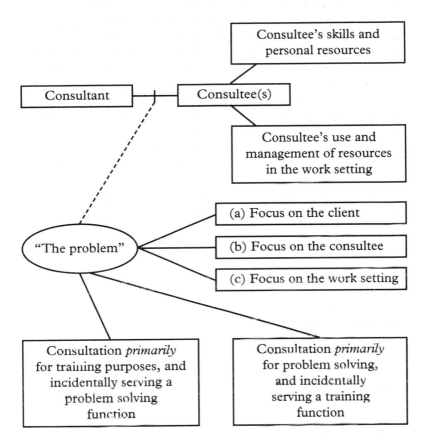

Areas of work in consultation

The theoretical bases for consultation

Consultative approaches draw on several theoretical models. The figure suggests the various topics on which consultation might focus as the problem solving exercise proceeds. First, there is the relationship between consultant and consultee, so that the science and art of interpersonal relationships and interpersonal skills are involved. However, it is important to recognise that consultation is an equal relationship in which consultant and consultee contribute their respective understanding and skills to problem solving. It is

121

essentially a joint exploration and negotiation, not about power but about how best to clarify an issue or problem and manage it.[12 47]

Second, there is the relation between the consultation and "the problem. So far, this has been discussed in terms of a patient's problem, so this dimension of the figure (a) is about clinical skills. We do not operate at peak efficiency all the time, especially when under pressure, and consultation, simply by creating a piece of focused space and time to take another look at a problem, can enable us to use our clinical skills more effectively. Nevertheless, the question in hand is not invariably a clinical one; a personal managerial issue is also a legitimate subject to consult about, and again in the relative calm, it is to be hoped, of a consultation it is possible to look again at such interprofessional individual or other individual or interpersonal matters that may concern the consultee (b).

Thus far, then, consultation is described in terms of helping to mobilise personal skills. But another possible focus for consultative work is that which is available, or missing, in the work setting (c)—for example facilities, staff, and such basics as time (and timetabling) and space. It is interesting how often what may look at first like a clinical problem, or a problem of personal skills, can emerge as a primarily organisational problem.[1–3] The process of systematic joint inquiry about the precise nature of the problem, and precisely what is needed, can come up with some surprising results: that a child care team, for example, does not have effective support or supervision, or that a department has a chaotic timetable, conflicting goals, or confused decision making and communication systems.

Part of the interest and challenge of consultative work is that the process of objective, shared inquiry into precisely what impedes and what enhances work may well lead into unexpected areas, whose practical implications and conceptual roots may be in, for example, social science, ethics, anthropology, or politics.[19 11–13] This can cause problems, as is discussed below.

Practical aspects of consultation

Consultation may therefore be centred on the consultee—that is, in terms of thinking through and reviewing how he or she has been dealing with a client or patient or a managerial, interprofessional issue that the consultee identifies—or the work setting. Of course, with mutual agreement, the focus can shift if that is appropriate.

Consultation has already been described as an activity in which the style of problem solving leads also to further learning. It is important to note that further learning can also be the *primary* purpose of a piece of consultative work—for example, child care teams may ask an outside consultant to help them develop their skills or the way they are organised, using day to day work issues as training material.

Consultation may be informal and *ad hoc*, for example a meeting over coffee, or in the way a referral or other inquiry is handled. It may involve two people, or a group, and may happen over a specific number of sessions or indefinitely.

Problems in consultation

Misunderstanding

If it is consultation as described here that is being sought or offered, that should be made clear. For example, if the transfer of responsibility to another clinician, or the transfer of care from one unit or ward to another (the term "disposal" is sometimes used) is wanted, it is annoying to be offered consultation instead. Such things happen, for example in intensive care areas.

Is consultation time consuming?

The question is rather to do with whose time is consumed, and when. Writing a referral note to a clinic, where a patient and parents are booked into a clinic some weeks hence, may take just a few minutes in terms of staff time. However, a detailed clinical assessment, perhaps after a wait of several weeks, may use many hours and turn out to be not necessary. A consultative response to referrals, or at least to some of them, may actually save time, enabling a more finely modulated response.[267] But it may not seem that way, and sometimes it may not be that way.

Consulting at the wrong level

It is an assumption of consultation that the consultee is at least potentially able, with help, to handle the matter in hand. However, if a problem looked like a clinical one (for example a registrar or staff nurse in difficulties over a case in an intensive care unit) but the answer lay in matters of policy (for example in terms of the medical or nursing training or supervision provided there), then the consultation would run into difficulties. Part of the skill of consultation is in checking that consultation is appropriate, with whom, and with what focus.

123

Straying into other territory

Consultation is something of a balancing act. It is not "support", or psychotherapy, or supervision, or about intervening in local politics or administration, and yet it approaches the edge of these areas. This is not simply a fine point of semantics. It is possible to get into real difficulty and may be professionally and legally hazardous if, for example, you believe you are offering consultation as defined here to a children's home but the local authority believes you are supervising its staff. Such muddles happen.

Confidentiality

Confidentiality is sometimes an unexpected problem. It is easier to preserve the confidentiality of a patient than that of an institution and its staff. There is also the problem of the consultant being unhappy about, say, practices in a children's home, or problems in the staff, and finding that consultation is making no impact. The expectation of consultation—that all participants will be responsible, within their roles and levels of expertise—is a help here rather than a hindrance, because if consultees cannot learn from consultation there should be a mutual agreement to end it. Perhaps supervision is needed instead. If a consultant discovered serious malpractice the same would apply, and if none of the consultees were willing to explain it to the appropriate authority the consultant, in a different role, might have to instead.

Excessive purity

Consultation needs to be reasonably clearly defined and its brief adhered to. At the same time it should be pragmatic and helpful, and should not become locked into a particular ideology. Thus the intention not to overlap with clinical work should not defy common sense if, for example, a doctor consulting to the staff of a children's home or a school suspected that a misbehaving child had a psychiatric problem. If there is an impasse over this or any other sort of problem there is an in-built solution: consult the consultees and review what you are doing; it is all grist to the consultative mill. Moreover, consultative and clinical approaches can be explicitly used together in a dual consultative–diagnostic approach, in which tasks are shared out as, for example, those for the social worker, those for the parents, those for the school, those for the clinician, and indeed those for the child. This is particularly helpful in child and adolescent psychiatric practice, where "who does what" can be contentious,[6-9 11] and in psychiatry generally, where "what is best" can be unclear[14] and deserves systematic consideration by all concerned.

Conclusion

In child and adolescent psychiatry, and I would suggest in related fields too, it is often not obvious which professional worker is the most appropriate for which type of presenting problem. Moreover, it often happens that several people are needed to work together, sometimes on an *ad hoc* basis, for a particular child's case. I doubt whether this could ever be worked out as part of a "grand design", or by computer. Consultation, as a collaborative skill all specialists could usefully have, offers a helpful way of clarifying who should do what with whom in a particular child's case, and it educates, and studies the field, as it proceeds.

This chapter is based on a talk given to the Congress of the European Society for Paediatrics held in Athens in October 1990.

1 Steinberg D. *Interprofessional consultation.* Oxford: Blackwell Scientific Publications, 1989.
2 Caplan G. *The theory and practice of mental health consultation.* London: Tavistock Publications, 1970.
3 Steinberg D, Hughes L. The emergence of work-centred issues in consultative work. *J Adolesc* 1987;**10**:309–16.
4 Conoley JC. *Consultation in schools: theory, research, procedures.* New York: Academic Press, 1981.
5 Gallesich J. *The profession and practice of consultation.* London: Jossey-Bass, 1982.
6 Steinberg D. *Basic adolescent psychiatry.* Oxford: Blackwell Scientific Publications, 1987.
7 Steinberg D. Management of crises and emergencies. In: Hsu LK, Hersen M, eds. *Recent developments in adolescent psychiatry.* New York: Wiley Interscience, 1989.
8 Steinberg D. Psychiatry: concepts, principles and practicalities. In: Brook CGD, ed. *Adolescent medicine.* Sevenoaks, Kent: Edward Arnold, 1993.
9 Steinberg D. *The clinical psychiatry of adolescence.* Chichester: Wiley, 1983.
10 Department of Health. *The Children Act 1989.* London: HMSO, 1989.
11 Steinberg D. Informed consent: consultation as a basis for collaboration between disciplines and between professionals and their patients. *Journal of Interprofessional Care* 1992;**6**:43–8.
12 Caplan G. *Principles of preventive psychiatry.* London: Tavistock Publications, 1964.
13 Trist E, Murray H, eds. *The social engagement of social science. I: The sociopsychological perspective.* London: Free Association Books, 1990.
14 Tyrer D, Steinberg D. *Models for mental disorder.* 2nd ed. Chichester: Wiley, 1993.

10. Psychiatric and paediatric liaison: development of a service

Shirley A Leslie

Introduction

This chapter describes the development of a psychiatric and paediatric liaison service. It highlights the changing needs and expectations of the service over the years and discusses how it can help clinical techniques. The service is based in a teaching hospital serving a local population but also containing several tertiary paediatric specialist units, and it has both clinical and teaching or junior medical training components.

The department of child psychiatry at Booth Hall Children's Hospital in north Manchester was founded in 1953. Although it has always been an integral part of the hospital, the fact that referrals came (initially) from a region containing over four million people meant that sometimes referrals from the hospital had to take their place in a very long queue.

Over the years the service has changed, staff have developed new skills, but new problems have arisen. A paediatric liaison service must remain flexible and responsive to new challenges. In my view, the best advice that has been given is to "be available, be practical, and be understandable".[1]

Availability

Being available meant that as a first priority the non-urgent outpatient waiting list was reduced to manageable proportions, even if that meant discouraging referrals from other districts, where there was a competent service, unless there was a definite request for a second opinion. One of my aims was, therefore, to encourage the development of district services throughout the

126

region, even though this meant that the number of consultants in child psychiatry at Booth Hall remained the same throughout the years (1968–89) that I was there. With the knowledge that a non-urgent referral could be dealt with reasonably promptly, a paediatrician would not be tempted to admit a child for a spurious reason to circumvent the waiting list.

Another measure to increase availability was the provision of a rota, whereby a member of the junior staff and a social worker would be able to assess all children admitted with self poisoning within 24 hours of them regaining consciousness. Urgent requests for help with a diagnostic problem in a child who is an inpatient are responded to within 48 hours, by either a consultant or senior registrar. A summary of the essential findings and recommendations is written in the paediatric case notes immediately after the assessment.

The apparent availability of the child psychiatrists was heightened by taking an active part in the division of paediatrics, attending paediatric postgraduate meetings, and by the simple but effective measure of having lunch with the other members of the medical staff.

Priorities

The way in which a paediatric liaison service is organised is liable to vary with the personal interests and expertise of the child psychiatrists concerned, and what is practicable in a given situation. There were several requests for combined ward rounds and joint clinics, but in the early years this was rarely done, mainly because of pressure of time.

Limited involvement in child abuse

At the beginning of the 1970s a decision was made not to get very involved in the management and treatment of families where there was suspected child abuse. At the time, the National Society for the Prevention of Cruelty to Children had set up a special unit in Manchester to offer a comprehensive service to these families, and it was thought that they would be able to offer more than we were able to. This was obviously different from the decision made in Oxford.[2] The rise in the recognition of sexual abuse in the 1980s and the increase in referrals of children with emotional and behavioural problems, where abuse was an important factor, forced us to reconsider this decision.

Self poisoning in adolescents

The sharp rise in the number of children admitted to hospital with self poisoning during the 1970s left us with no option but to respond promptly and effectively. It was our policy that no child should leave the hospital without themselves being seen by the doctor who would be responsible for following them up. A member of the child's family would also be seen, before the child was discharged, to encourage future involvement with the child psychiatric team if this was thought to be necessary.[3]

Responding to changing needs and expectations

Between these extremes of full involvement in what is commonly regarded as the true province of the psychiatrist, as with attempted suicide, and disengagement from what could be seen as exclusively the province of the social worker and paediatrician, as with physical child abuse, there remained the decision about how best to respond to other requests for help. These were mainly requests for assistance with the diagnosis of a sick child, help in the management of the common disorders of childhood that are known to have a psychological component, and referrals of children with prolonged and sometimes disabling disorders such as epilepsy, diabetes, asthma, and cystic fibrosis.

Staff on the burns and neurosurgical units also needed support and guidance in the best ways to help families whose children had been severely injured. Likewise, at a later stage, staff on the intensive care unit felt in need of training over how best to cope with their own feelings about being constantly in touch with dying children and their families.

The child psychiatrist needed to be able to provide help to the individual child and to his or her carers. There was also a need to teach staff how to recognise a psychological problem and how to become more aware of their own reactions in stressful situations.

Paediatricians and their supporting staff needed to know how to handle a referral to a child psychiatrist or psychologist and how to improve their ability to treat common problems so that some referrals are possibly no longer necessary.

Requests for help with diagnosis

The referral process

Referrals for help with a diagnosis remain the principal component of our liaison service. This type of referral is best carried out at senior level and it is essential that the paediatrician or senior registrar discuss the referral with the parents and the child, if old enough, beforehand.

Psychiatry still carries a stigma in the mind of the average person and it is here that the paediatrician's trust in the psychiatrist to whom he or she is going to refer is vital. An explanation that anxieties can sometimes give rise to pain that is genuinely felt should dispel the notion that the child is a liar or a fraud.

Similarly, it is important to help parents to see that referral to a child psychiatrist does not necessarily mean that their child is mentally ill or that the report will form part of a child's school record. As far as the child is concerned, the doctor is one who talks to children about worries and problems. Children are encouraged to know that no painful procedures, such as injections, will be given.

The psychiatric assessment

The process of psychiatric interviewing is of necessity detailed and should not be rushed. As well as one or two interviews with the child, there must be at least one with a parent, preferably both. Psychiatrists are trained to make a positive psychiatric diagnosis and not to rely solely on the absence of physiological signs. With children, this will mean an understanding of the dynamics of the

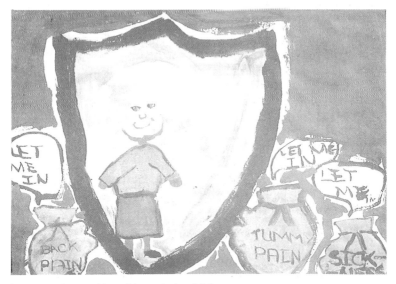

Stress can be manifested by pain in children

family and whether or not a symptom is being used for a secondary gain.[45]

Prompt and confident psychiatric diagnosis may spare a child unnecessary investigative procedures and shorten the period of disability.[6] When the issues are less clear, paediatrician and child psychiatrist may continue to work closely together, perhaps during an inpatient assessment, either in a paediatric ward or in a child psychiatric inpatient unit.

Requests for help with common disorders

Enuresis

Referrals of children with enuresis, encopresis, and sleep disorders were very common 20 years ago. The improvements in available treatment techniques have meant that only the most intractable now reach a child psychiatric clinic. Children with enuresis, when they are thought not to have a physical problem, are either dealt with in primary care or their treatment programme is supervised by a clinical psychologist. This is entirely appropriate as children with monosymptomatic enuresis should not be considered to have a psychiatric disorder.[7]

Encopresis

Encopresis that is not associated with any physical disorder is sometimes associated with other behaviour problems and may warrant a full psychiatric assessment. Nevertheless, many cases can be dealt with symptomatically, especially those thought to be due to the withholding of faeces, for whatever reason. Behavioural treatments have proved the most effective and can be administered by a psychologist or a suitably trained community nurse, though most studies have shown that a prolonged follow up is essential.[8]

Sleeping problems

The improvement in methods of helping the parents of young children with sleeping problems[9] has meant that health visitors now feel more competent to treat these disorders in primary care. In some areas sleep clinics have been established to give support and advice to parents with unusually fretful and wakeful children.

One of my priorities over the years was to help health visitors to understand the factors that often underlie some of the common behavioural problems in young children and some basic principles for tackling them.[10]

Children with disabling disorders

The referral of children who are having a particular problem in coming to terms with some aspect of a chronic illness or handicap is often an appropriate referral to a child psychiatric service. For instance the presence of family conflict and the dissatisfaction of a mother with her marriage has been shown to relate to poor diabetic control in a child with that disorder.[11] Likewise, family problems may exacerbate the severity of symptoms in some asthmatic children.[12]

Adolescents also become extremely sensitive about physical disfigurements that previously they had seemed to take in their stride. Similar problems are experienced by epileptic children. The problems may manifest themselves in different ways: depression, school avoidance, or behavioural change. Much will depend on what importance the disease process or handicap has for the child and his or her family.[13 14]

Although services now exist for most of these groups, providing peer support for children and their parents, some children benefit from individual supportive psychotherapy and others from family therapy. Most can be dealt with in the main outpatient service. Joint clinics can be helpful, especially if a clinic is set aside where patients who both a paediatrician and child psychiatrist have in common can be seen by both together, but we do not have these very often.

Box 1—Indications for psychiatric–paediatric liaison

Diagnosing a psychiatric disorder contributing to physical illness
Self poisoning
The more severe forms of common problems: enuresis,
    encopresis, sleep disorders
Sexual abuse
Children with disabling physical disorders
Supporting staff working in stressful units (for example, coping
    with the dying child).

Services to regional specialist units

At Booth Hall there are regional services for the treatment of burns, a renal dialysis unit, and departments of neurosurgery and neurology. Because of the severity of the children's problems and the way in which their behaviours often caused a great deal of anxiety to the nursing staff, these units were the first to demand, and for some of the time to get, their own direct liaison with either a child psychiatrist or a clinical psychologist.

Burns unit

The direct liaison provided by a clinical psychologist to the burns unit enables the staff to see the trauma as affecting the whole family and not only the child patient. Supporting the family's feelings of guilt and helplessness is as important as encouraging the child to come to terms with his or her disfigurement.[15] Referrals to the child psychiatrist are then only made when a child was severely behaviourally disturbed, in a toxic confusional state, or unusually depressed and withdrawn.

Neurosurgical unit

Similarly, the neurosurgical unit has a clinical psychologist with a sessional attachment, which means that the common sequelae of children with head injuries are clearly undertsood by the staff and the expected difficulties communicated to both the parents and the child's school teachers on discharge. The children who are referred to child psychiatry usually have very severe injuries or a pre-existing psychiatric disorder, or both.

Renal unit

My child psychiatry colleague undertook to have a liaison role with the renal unit. She was able to attend ward meetings and became an important member of the team. Psychiatric assessment of the children shows that more definite psychological difficulties occurs in the children with the most severe illness. However, psychiatric disturbance is again related to stress in the family and compliance with drug treatment.[16]

Neurology unit

A major part of our liaison work is in the neurology department. It is common practice for the neurologist to discuss a case with a psychiatrist before admission when a combined assessment is thought to be important. The agreement of suitable dates for the child's admission is then possible. Frequently such patients are treated jointly on the medical ward.[17]

Follow up

Most of these referrals from the specialist units involve children who live outside the district. Follow up is therefore sometimes difficult, though parents are often prepared to travel considerable distances at their own expense. It is, however, rarely thought appropriate to refer children to the local child psychiatric service when it has not been involved in any of the inpatient treatment. We suspect that such referrals would not be taken up by the families. This has major staffing implications for specialised teaching units who wish to encourage a closer child psychiatric liaison.

Teaching

The essence of good teaching is to make the subject understandable. Psychiatrists are well known for using jargon only understood by the initiated. Writing reports and letters in a way that makes sense to the average intelligent doctor is a good way of teaching a subject and should not be underestimated. Whenever possible our department's assessment and recommendations for treatment are put in letter form addressed to the paediatrician or relevant consultant and a copy sent to the family doctor.

Postgraduate

Attending clinical meetings and participating in postgraduate training in paediatrics is a regular part of our work. Our monthly child psychiatric case conference is held in the postgraduate centre and is available to all. From time to time we are also able to suggest speakers for day conferences on such themes as the care of the dying child.

Undergraduate

The clinical teaching of child psychiatry to undergraduates takes place during their paediatric placement.[18] As well as attending outpatient clinics and seeing videotaped interviews with child psychiatric patients they also attend weekly seminars, taken by the senior staff, in which they are asked to present cases they have seen. Four of the students are asked to present a paediatric case from a psychosocial point of view. Most have difficulty with the concept at first, as they have the patients neatly compartmentalised into paediatric and psychiatric.

The aim is to help them to look at such issues as how a family of a child with a life threatening disease copes or why a baby with a chest infection has not been visited. Sometimes the group is stimulated to look at deeper issues such as how they feel about the death of a child and how they would help a family come to terms with the birth of a handicapped child.

Box 2—Therapeutic strategies in psychiatric–paediatric liaison

Availability: short waiting list at the child psychiatric clinic
rota for emergency work
Making a positive psychiatric diagnosis
Occasional joint psychiatric and paediatric clinics
Development of special links by psychiatrists with specific units, for example neurological or other tertiary paediatric units
Psychiatrists' attendance at paediatric meetings
Teaching paediatric postgraduates and undergraduates during their paediatric training.

Conclusion

This account of the development of a paediatric liaison service to a specialist children's hospital in north Manchester does not detail every kind of case we saw. We estimated that about 25% of our referrals came from our own hospital. Because of our commitments to more than one district service and a supradistrict child psychiatric inpatient unit our services were inevitably stretched.

As the service has developed clinical psychologists have become able to take on the direct liaison with some specialist units, thereby helping the nursing staff to have a better understanding of the emotional and behavioural problems of their patients. Likewise the outcome of a regular clinic between one of the paediatric surgeons and a child psychiatrist was the establishment of a district nursing service for children with encopresis. It is essential that in this type of service all disciplines can refer to each other and that communication between them is easy. The welfare of the child is more important than keeping to rigid professional boundaries. To a large extent a service will develop according to the resources available.

There are many advantages to child psychiatrists in being part of a paediatric service. We are kept up to date in the paediatric specialty and we hope that our frequent exposure to the influence of paediatricians prevents us from becoming too set in our ways or inclined to make extravagant claims for our specialty.

In return, we hope that paediatrics gains from our insistence on seeing children and their disease or handicap in the context of their level of understanding, their life experience, and their family situation. As our knowledge base has increased, and treatment techniques have become more specific, we hope that a basic understanding of our specialty will be a part of every paediatrician's training.

The picture in this chapter is reproduced with permission from the Victoria and Albert museum.

1 Rothenberg MB. Child psychiatry–paediatric consultation liaison services in the hospital setting. *Gen Hosp Psychiatry* 1979;1:281–6.
2 Lynch M, Robertson J. *Consequences of child abuse.* London: Academic Press, 1982.
3 Kerfoot M. Deliberate self poisoning in childhood and early adolescence. *J Child Psychol Psychiatry* 1988;29:335–44.
4 Stone FH. *Psychiatry and the paediatrician.* London: Butterworths, 1975:19–32.
5 Mrazek D. Child psychiatric consultation and liaison to paediatrics. In Rutter M, Hersov L, eds. *Child and adolescent psychiatry. Modern approaches.* Oxford: Blackwell, 1985:888–9.
6 Dubowitz V, Hersov L. Management of children with non-organic (hysterical) disorders of motor function. *Dev Med Child Neurol* 1976;18:358–68.
7 Graham P. Enuresis: a child psychiatrist's approach. In: Kolvin I, MacKeith RC, Meadow SR, eds. *Bladder control and enuresis. Clinics in developmental medicine 48/49.* London: Heinemann/Spastics International Medical Publications. 1973:276–80.
8 Hersov L. Faecal soiling. In: Rutter M, Hersov L, eds. *Child and adolescent psychiatry. Modern approaches.* Oxford: Blackwell, 1985:482–9.
9 Douglas J, Richman N *My child won't sleep.* Harmondsworth: Penguin Handbooks, 1984.
10 Lask B. *Children's problems: A parent's guide to understanding and tackling them.* London: Dunitz, 1985.
11 Marteau TM, Bloch S, Baum JD. Family life and diabetic control. *J Child Psychol Psychiatry* 1987;28:823–34.
12 Mrazek DA. Childhood asthma: two central questions for child psychiatry. *J Child Psychol Psychiatry* 1986;27:1–5.
13 Taylor DC. The components of sickness: diseases illnesses and predicaments. In: Apley J, Ounsted C, eds. *One child.* London: Heinemann/Spastics International Medical Publications, 1982:1–13.
14 Hoare J. Children with epilepsy and their families. *J Child Psychol Psychiatry* 1987;28:651–5.
15 Rivlin E. The psychological trauma and management of severe burns in children and adolescents. *Br J Hosp Med* 1988;40:210–5.
16 Garralda ME, Jameson RA, Reynolds JM, Postlethwaite RJ. Psychiatric adjustment in children with chronic renal failure. *J Child Psychol Psychiatry* 1988;29:79–90.
17 Leslie SA. The diagnosis and treatment of hysterical conversion reactions. *Arch Dis Child* 1988;63:506–11.
18 Garralda ME. Teaching child psychiatry to medical students: students feedback. *Psychiatric Bulletin* 1984;8:171–2.

11. Dealing with the courts and parenting breakdown

Claire Sturge

The resolution of disputes, problems, and uncertainties through the court system, as well as safeguarding the interests of the child, can actually promote these and be therapeutic. I use here therapeutic in the sense of an agent of positive change, ultimately for the child concerned.

Until now this has been best exemplified in the High Courts. One of the main challenges of the Children Act 1989 is whether this tool of positive intervention can be used as constructively and to the full in the lower courts and even transferred out into the community in precourt or no court situations.

Civil court proceedings concerning children and adolescents will almost always be about some form of parenting breakdown.

The purpose of this chapter is threefold: (a) to explore why child health specialists, particularly child psychiatrists, have come to be involved in the assessment of parenting breakdown and what relevant or essential skills they bring to the decision making process; (b) to demystify court proceedings by clarifying and simplifying them; and (c) to identify the constructive elements of court processes so that readers can determine how they can have a role in these and extend them to other situations.

The interrelation of the courts and child health specialists

Paediatricians and child psychiatrists are increasingly being asked to write reports for court—as expert rather than evidential witnesses—and this is likely to increase further with the Children Act 1989 and its emphasis on multidisciplinary assessment.

Courts are clearly mandated to concern themselves with the physical and emotional well being of children. Paediatric assessment, uniquely in medicine, has already moved to considering all aspects of a child's health, including the emotional adjustment and development. While a child psychiatrist may be the one assessing emotional adjustment in detail, the paediatrician has important contributions to make.

What physical abuse did for the paediatrician, sexual abuse has done for the child psychiatrist. The "discovery" of physical child abuse in the 1950s gradually brought paediatricians into a central role in court proceedings, and the "discovery" of child sexual abuse in the 1980s brought child psychiatrists into the arena. Awareness of sexual abuse and the type of evidence child psychiatrists were giving about its sequelae brought into focus the fact that the most serious and longer lasting effects of *any* abuse are the result of the emotional component of that abuse. We can expect that with this third new awareness, more cases will be brought under the sole category of emotional abuse.

This chain highlighting emotional abuse brings parenting as a whole under scrutiny: emotional abuse becomes equated with gross parenting failure on an emotional level or, put another way, a gross failure to meet a child's psychological needs for his or her healthy emotional development. (Parenting breakdown can, of course, involve other forms of abuse, physical or sexual, but will include an emotional component.)

This recognition has led to examination of how parenting can be analysed, what are its components, and how these can be assessed or measured. There is some agreement on its components but very little on how to measure or assess these systematically.

Parenting assessment

The components are best extracted by considering a child's basic needs (see box 1).

How to assess these needs

There are various approaches for assessing needs—for example, the social services assessment pack[3] and the National Children's Bureau child protection pack.[4] There are assessments based almost entirely on interactional processes—for example those described by Reder,[5] Cox et al,[6] Dowdney et al,[7] and Bentovim and Gilmour.[8] Questionnaires, checklists, rating scales, and other instruments are of limited value in individual cases. For a compendium

> ### Box 1—Parenting assessment: the child's basic needs
>
> Security/safety:
> *Safety*: food, warmth, clothing, etc and home, car, road, personal safety
> *Security*: sense of safety necessary for security; stability and consistency of
>   care givers, care itself, discipline, and boundaries. Mutual trust. Sense
>   of being listened to and good channels of communication. Perception of
>   parents as strong, able to cope, being in control, responsive
>
> Belongingness:
> Continuity of care givers. Clear identity, for example, names, roots,
>   culture. Sense of permanence. Personal or individual space and
>   possessions
>
> Self actualisation/identity development:
> Child treated as special and unique. Child seen as separate from parent by
>   the parent(s) (distinction of needs). Perceptiveness of child's
>   individuality and particular needs. Lack of intrusiveness
>
> Praise/esteem:
> Meeting of child's need for esteem and praise. Expression of warmth and
>   positive feelings, absence of hostility. Appropriate positive
>   reinforcement. Valuing the child's differentness
>
> New experience/knowledge:
> Encouragement of learning, extending new experiences and independence
> Giving child sense of responsibility for his/her actions and for their
>   impact on others.

Modified from Kellmer Pringle and Maslow.[12]

of these see the *Handbook of Family Measurement Techniques*.[9]
Semistructured interviews used in research may have a place.[10]

I take a more pragmatic approach by firstly, gathering information (from social services, schools, paediatricians, foster carers, etc) and secondly, making my own assessment of parenting through (a) direct discussions with the parent(s), (b) assessment of the child(ren) to assess their development and particular needs, and (c) observations of interactions between child(ren) and parents. In this way, I attempt to cover all the components of parenting listed above, the details of which vary greatly with age. I pay particular attention to positive remarks about the child, criticism, and indications of warmth or hostility, all of which have been consistently shown to be assessable in a fairly reliable way and to relate to quality of parenting.[11] The parent(s) own experience of parenting is important. In situations of breakdown, my experience is that it has invariably been one of insecure or preoccupied type (see Crowell and Feldman[12]).

Having made an initial formulation considering all the components of the parenting needs, I structure observations of interactions between child(ren) and parents to target particular areas where problems may lie. If major problems are identified in this way then assessment of the parent's or parents' ability to change must follow.

Assessing ability to change

Prerequisites for change include:
● Acknowledgement of some responsibility for current situation, for example, child being in care.
● Acceptance that there is a need for change and that the parents themselves need to change.
● Acceptance of need for help in this.
● Child should not be used systematically as a scapegoat.

Capacity to change may be assessed by:
● History of change or lack of change over time
● History of cooperativeness and openness with "helping" professions
● Ability to reflect during assessment
● Carry over of content of discussion from one assessment meeting to another, indicating change of attitude
● Tasks can be set to assess this more directly: they can be (i) within session or between session, (ii) directly or indirectly related to problems, and (iii) passive or active
● Personality, illness, and level of intelligence issues are also important factors in ability to change.

For a more comprehensive approach and model see Protchasha and Di Clemente, Bentovim *et al*, and Jones.[13-15] The parent–child game[16] is an interesting new approach to assessing parents' ability to improve on interactional skills.

Predictions about change are based on all of the above and the input considered necessary to support change.

Exploring alternatives

There needs to be a careful look at alternatives: possibilities for solutions within family or extended family, the resources available for support or therapy, and how the best possible environment for change can be created. Again this is likely to require a collaborative effort, with everyone in the multiagency network exploring their resources and offering their knowledge of resources available elsewhere.

Under the Children Act 1989, in effect, every request for a full order will be thrown out where it cannot be shown that every avenue has been explored for ways to keep the family together. Under the Children Act 1989 it should be possible to undertake the whole assessment that I have described long before, or without any, recourse to court.

The child psychiatrist's contribution

Child psychiatrists have skills in all areas relating to assessing parenting and the ability to change. Of particular relevance are the following:

● A multiaxial approach to classification, looking at the child in terms of psychiatric, cognitive, developmental, and biological functioning and social situation.

● Expertise in family psychiatry resulting from family centred work and the large body of knowledge on family functioning from the different schools of family therapy.

● Knowledge of child development.

● Knowledge about child temperament and its interactional importance.[17]

● Knowledge of adult psychiatry and, from this, knowledge about what parenting functions are likely to be impaired in a parent with a psychiatric or personality disorder. The child psychiatrist will also have some knowledge about treatment and prognosis that will be very important in decisions about the child and has easy access to adult psychiatrists to consult over this.

● A "scientific" approach. Medically trained practitioners do have particular skills to offer in these decision making processes, not simply by virtue of their knowledge base but also as the result of their particular and rigorous training involving the Socratean approach, an emphasis on cause and effect, pros and cons, and a healthy scepticism, particularly in examining evidence.

We are disciplined to think in terms of "What evidence do I have for making that statement?" and "On what am I basing my opinion?" This approach, which is not so highly developed in other disciplines, together with the knowledge already outlined, will be particularly useful to courts where the issue is centred on whether the harm the child has suffered, or may suffer, is significant (a central concept in the Children Act 1989).

Prediction about the child's future is a most difficult and onerous task because far reaching decisions about the child may be based on it. In my opinion, this task falls most appropriately to the child psychiatrist. The child psychiatrist can formulate the problems on a multiaxial basis and base a prognosis on this. The very fact of childhood involves central concepts concerned with the child as a developing being with considerable potential for change, and all the variables of the child's past experience, temperament, present state, and future environment impinge on this. Attempts can be made, for example, to answer questions about the likely outcome in terms of emotional and behavioural adjustment of a sexually abused child exhibiting traumatised behaviours depending on whether she or he remains with the parent or is put in care and whether therapy is or is not offered. Child psychiatrists also have a contribution to make in considering transcultural issues in placement decisions, when the relative importance of identity development against other development needs must be weighed.

Clearly where there is psychiatric disturbance, the child psychiatrist has an important contribution to make. Particularly difficult cases involve children with an innate problem, for example autism, where a parent's care is in question and the question, under the Children Act 1989, is whether another parent with such a child would be making a better job of it.

Box 2 summarises the common contexts of parenting breakdown, and box 3 lists some of the court mechanisms for dealing with them.

Court decisions

For courts to make decisions, the following are necessary. (1) Identifying the central issue(s) and the questions that need to be answered for a decision to be made. (2) Requiring all parties to justify their actions and criticisms with evidence. (3) Requiring that the evidence necessary to answer the central questions is produced. (4) Exploring alternatives, particularly that of no court order.

In addition, the courts can be particularly useful in:

- Ensuring very thorough assessment.
- Confronting families with what is at stake—that is, possible loss of the care of a child.
- Making orders compelling compliance where a parent's own

Box 2—Parenting breakdown	
Problem/concern	*Main focus for assessment in addition to parenting*
Physical abuse	Paediatric assessment: risk to health and life. Emotional damage
Sexual abuse	Non-abusing parent's ability to support and protect child. Child's emotional state and needs, treatment needs
Failure to thrive; physical deprivation	Paediatric assessment
Emotional abuse, emotional deprivation	Child's emotional state and needs, treatment needs
Munchausen syndrome by proxy	Paediatric assessment: risk to health and life. Psychiatric assessment of parent
Parental mental disorder: mental illness, personality disorder, substance abuse, mental handicap	Psychiatric/psychology assessment with particular reference to ability to make responsible decisions and progress
Beyond control: usually adolescents	Assessment of youngster's needs

motivation is insufficient to result in change. This is, of course, not always successful.[18]

● Clearly defining criteria for measuring change on which future decisions will be based.

● Balancing the power between any individual—for example, a parent—and an agency such as social services. Redressing the balance between parties can in itself be therapeutic and is less likely to occur when a case is handled entirely within one agency.

The whole process should be one of clarifying issues and identifying the most objective means of answering questions in relation to them.

The court is attempting to choose the least detrimental option, in the best interests of the child. In practice, it can decide where the child lives, who has day to day and other responsibilities, details of contact with others, and treatment needs. Decisions directly affecting adults are much more limited, particularly in the lower courts.

The party initiating proceedings—for medical practitioners this is usually social services or a parent—initiates this process by deciding what order they are seeking and on what grounds. The initiating party must then seek to produce evidence to support those grounds. The more experienced the initiating solicitor the

> ## Box 3—Courts: civil proceedings concerning children and adolescents in magistrates and county courts and High Courts
>
> | Issues | Parties | Range of orders or directions |
> | --- | --- | --- |
> | Parenting breakdown including abuse and being beyond parental control | Social services and others—for example, grandparents | Residence, contact, supervision and care orders, specific directions |
> | School non-attendance | Education authority, parents | Education supervision order |
> | Marital breakdown | Between parents | Residence orders, specific issues, contact (care, control custody, and access are all gone) |
> | Welfare and consent issues such as child abduction, treatment refusal | Any | Wardship with its inherent powers, including children act orders (High Court) |
> | Challenges about statutory services—for example, services to a child "in need" | Any: particularly parents versus education, social services, or health authorities | Judicial review: decisions are binding on parties |

better the questions will be that are asked to elicit information and evidence.

I have been involved in many cases, at the county court or High Court level, where in effect the dispute is between the parent and a social services department where the parent, for a variety of reasons (often containing a large antiauthoritarian element), has completely fallen out with the social services department and a hostile relationship exists on both sides. The parent's failure to cooperate is then used as further evidence of their lack of responsibility and ability to change.

A court can look at this objectively and lean on social services departments, if necessary, to change the social worker or use an independent agency. Alternatively, if the lack of cooperation is deemed appreciable in terms of the child's interest, a court can make this explicit to the parent, laying down what cooperation the court expects if an order in the parent's favour is to be considered. I have seen very constructive work become possible with the most intransigent parents in this situation (see Familaro et al[18]). Of course, it is theoretically possible for this to be achieved by other means, for example the fashionable contracts. These, however, have no legal status and mean social services have "no teeth" without the backup of a court. Nor do they deal with the power imbalance referred to above (see Wolff et al[19]).

A vignette

This is a greatly simplified example. A social services department wishes to seek a care order as a result of a mother being found on two occasions drunk and incapable when in charge of her three children aged under 5 years, one of whom actually went missing. The children are currently on an interim care order, in foster care. The middle child, a boy aged 3, uses no expressive language.

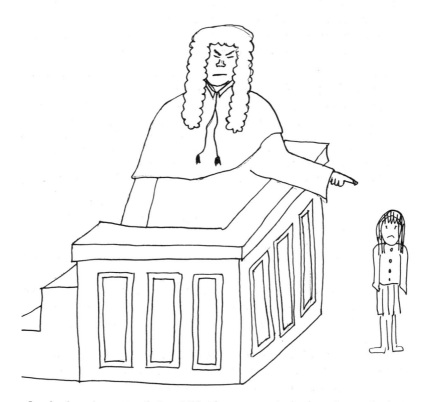

In the best interests of the child, the court attempts to choose the least detrimental option

The issue would be: is this mother able to parent responsibly? The questions would be: what are the mother's parenting capacities? to what degree are these affected by drink? what is the prognosis as regards her drinking? how have the children been affected? is the 3 year old's language problem innate or the result of disturbed emotional development? is there any way of ensuring these children's safety without removing them? is there any input that would enable this mother to fulfill her responsibilities?

The social worker involved with the case may have much of this information, but for two reasons additional outside expertise is likely to be required. (1) Social workers do not present their evidence in an "expert" fashion addressing issues in a systematic manner. This is exacerbated by their own solicitors treating them as inexpert by not requiring reports to answer specific questions but by requiring sworn affidavits, usually of a narrative type, for example on date X I went to the house and found Y. Opinions are not encouraged. (2) The social services department needs to call in outside expertise in areas in which they have little or none. Requirements for the assessment are shown in box 4.

Box 4—Requirements for an assessment

Full assessment: area to be assessed	*By whom*
Children's health and physical and emotional development	Social services, child health specialist, child psychiatrist
The mother's own history Stresses on the mother	Social services and child health professionals
The mother's parenting abilities Mother's ability to change	Social services, child psychiatrist, clinical child psychologist, or combination of these
Mother's mental state, alcohol problem and its prognosis	Adult psychiatry

---

As can be seen, a collaborative effort is required and there will be important inputs from the health visitor, general practitioner, nursery if applicable, and others who know the mother and children.

The concept of multidisciplinary assessment in addressing the needs of children is central to the new Children Act. The social services department usually initiates and coordinates such multi-disciplinary assessments, including child assessment orders (in which the courts can control the nature of the assessment).

Though child psychiatrist may, for the present, be the group able to contribute most comprehensively to parenting assessment, their numbers are too few to be involved in all cases. Others, particularly clinical psychologists specialising in children, have a great deal to offer.

I do believe that child psychiatrists' skills are essential in certain complex situations:

● Where the child has a pronounced psychiatric disorder.

● Where a child's or adolescent's allegations are subject to doubt because of contradications, inconsistencies, clearly fanciful parts, or a history of lying or fantasising. (The whole area of how to approach the validation of allegations is a subject in itself.)

● Where the parent has a pronounced psychiatric disorder.

● Where there is a need to interpret the meaning of a child's behaviour, for example, emotional reactions to contact with a parent or non-verbal behaviours such as play or acting out.

● Where there is a need to determine prognosis about a child's disorder.

● Where there is a Munchausen's by proxy type of syndrome in which, for example, a parent's overwhelming belief that a child has been sexually abused, in the absence of any evidence, becomes in itself, abusive.

Tips

A question to be considered when you become involved in court proceedings is: who is instructing you? If this is your own local authority, the assessment is under your NHS contract, the writing of a report for court or attendance at court is section 2 work. If it is the local authority, check whether a *guardian ad litem* has been appointed. If so, insist he or she is consulted about social services instructing you. If the guardian approves your doing the assessment this will avoid duplication—important for the child but also in order to conserve our own overstretched resources. If the guardian or a private solicitor is instructing you all the work will be section 2 work and usually be paid out of legal aid monies which are very restricting. Negotiating what can be done for a specified sum can be very time consuming. Ethically this can be difficult—is half an assessment better than none?

Whoever is instructing you, the most important thing, and that which will determine the quality of the whole process, is the questions you are asked to answer. Make sure these questions are

146

entirely open—that is, not "should this mother ever see her children again?" but "what is your opinion on future contact between mother and children?" It is well worth the investment of time in getting questions clarified. If I get very biased questions, particularly from a private solicitor, this may determine me against taking the case.

Always get prior agreement to your report going to all parties. Your report is by definition unbiased but can be suppressed by the instructing solicitor. Occasionally I even go as far as sending a copy to the clerk of the court.

If the request comes from your local authority, consider whether you will be able to act in a sufficiently independent way. It can be very difficult to implicitly criticise one's local department or make costly recommendations and then continue working with the department day to day.

Reports usually need to be long, when difficult decisions are involved, to include all the evidence and alternative arguments. The summary and recommendations should be short. The recommendations, though most attention is paid to them, are the least important as our job is to give the court all the necessary information on which to base its decisions. My reports vary from five to 50 pages (the latter if there are several children and many possible outcomes).

It is worth forging links with the local courts, for example expressing a wish to meet the magistrates and the borough solicitors. I am usually not called in the lower courts, but if I am the borough solicitors and the courts do everything in their power to make this as convenient as possible.

Child Psychiatry and the Law is a most useful reference book when involved in court work.[20]

General comment

I hope this chapter has made clear that, by the very process of clarification and careful, objective assessment together with their innate authority, courts can have a very positive effect in furthering children's interests. For this reason, while welcoming the Children Act as the most exciting step taken in children's interests in my working lifetime, I am concerned about the inevitable impact of the act in relation to court proceedings.

(1) Wardship has virtually disappeared and in particular I believe this deprives parents (and therefore the child) of the

highest level of judicial consideration where a parent may be overpowered in a situation of conflict with a statutory body.

(2) There will be a downwards movement in terms of the level of court. All cases will start in the Family Proceedings Courts and most will stay there. We have yet to see how easy it is to get the more complex cases moved up to higher courts. My knowledge of magistrates and their training, and the solicitors and barristers involved in these lower proceedings makes me very concerned that children will lose out because of lesser expertise. Complexity will be gauged by the intensity of the "war"—that is, the number of affidavits—rather than on the actual wisdom required to decide a multi-issue situation for a child.

The important thing is to be aware of, and to address, these issues. Any party can apply to the registrar for a transfer of court, and the health authority may in future see cause to make itself a party more frequently.

(3) My third concern relevant to this chapter is the concept of theoretically everextending parental responsibility for children so that they can have multiple "parents". Though useful for adults in underlining concepts of responsibilities rather than rights, I believe it will be confusing for children and their need for clarity and security.

(4) My fourth major concern is that without the high court there is no court review procedure. Once a child is in care, there is no process that allows a court to review how social services is progressing the case, for example no curb on delays, say, in finding a long term placement. Social services may welcome this, I do not. This also denies magistrates the opportunity to learn from the experience of seeing how court decisions turn out. (Scottish law allows for this.)

(5) My fifth concern relates to problems that are likely to result from overstretched resources within all the agencies. This will affect (a) assessment in general, and (b) the provision of alternatives. *Assessments*: there is likely to be a conscious or unconscious resistance to take on in depth assessment work. I am continually struck by how even the consideration of court proceedings, and certainly actual court proceedings, can transform a case and get movement and outcomes not originally considered possible—as a result of the processes I have described of clarifying issues and trying to answer questions connected with these issues. In addition, the particular skills of the legal profession in the process of clarification and objective assessment will not be available if legal

proceedings are not being considered. *The provision of alternatives*: with the lack of financial resource in social services and limited treatment facilities within the health authority and social services, some families are likely to be treated unfairly. If intensive treatment is not available then local authority care may be the only alternative where there are major parenting problems. We are often faced with the dilemma of whether to recommend an approach to enable change when we know that the resource is not available through the local health authority or social services and may need to be paid for in the independent sector. This is a particular problem when working with our own local authority.

I look forward positively to a future in which we can continue to develop ways of working with the courts that make use of the very constructive processes that I have outlined and in which we all learn to take those processes of assessment and intervention, which can also be productive outside the legal framework, into our interagency work.

I find this type of work often to be doubly satisfying: it is intellectually the most challenging I undertake and in terms of altering children's lives for the better often the most effective input I can have.

Child and family legislation in Scotland, Northern Ireland, and the Republic of Ireland

The legal arrangements for handling child care proceedings are very different from in England and Wales, although the basic philosophy is similar.

In Scotland, the main and considerable difference is the system of children's hearings. These already incorporate many features of the Children Act 1989, for example, children are able to take an active part and families are closely involved. It has a specialist element that many hope to see eventually in England and Wales and the advantage of an informal, non-adversarial system, the combining of all children's proceedings (criminal and civil), and an inbuilt review system. See part III of the Social Work (Scotland) Act 1968 which embroidered the recommendations of the Kilbrandon report.

In the Republic of Ireland new children's legislation was enacted in July 1991. The Child Care Act 1991 is currently being implemented, and it is expected that this process will be completed by 1996/7. The new legislation brings a major shift in attitudes to child welfare, with the new emphasis being placed on the "best interest of the child". The community care programmes in the local health boards are charged with the responsibility of promoting the welfare of children in their areas. To this end, the act lays great stress on prevention programmes and family support services. The introduction of supervision orders as an alternative to the removal of children from home, and the proposal to provide for a *guardian ad litem* system, are but two indicators of the new "child centred" approach. The main thrust of the legislation is broadly in line with the UK Children Act 1989.

In Northern Ireland a new Children Order (Northern Ireland) is being prepared. It is expected to be ready by the autumn of 1993 and will be very similar to the UK Children Act 1989. Until then, the Children and Young Persons Act 1968 applies, which is similar to the 1969 act in England and Wales for young people.

1 Kellmer Pringle M. *The needs of children.* London: Hutchinson, 1975.
2 Maslow AH. *Motivation and personality.* New York: Harper and Row, 1954.
3 Department of Health. *Protecting children: a guide for social workers undertaking a comprehensive assessment.* London: HMSO, 1988.
4 National Children's Bureau. Significant harm and its treatment. *Child protection: a training and practice resource pack for work under the Children Act, 1989.* London: NCB, 1991.
5 Reder P, Lucey C. The assessment of parenting: some interactional considerations. *Psychiatric Bulletin* 1991;**15**:347–8.
6 Cox AD, Pound A, Mills M, Puckering C, Owen AL. Evaluation of a home visiting and befriending scheme for young mothers: Newpin. *J R Soc Med* 1991;**84**:17–20.
7 Dowdney L, Skuse D, Rutter M, Mtazek D. Parenting qualities: concepts, measures and origins. In: Stevenson JE, ed. *Recent research in developmental psychopathology.* Pergamon, 1985:19–42.
8 Bentovim A, Gilmour L. A family therapy interactional approach to decision making in child care, custody and access cases. *Journal of Family Therapy* 1981;**1**:65–77.
9 Touliatos J, ed. *Handbook of family measurement techniques.* Newbury Park, California: Sage, 1990.
10 Rutter M, Quinton D, Liddle C. Parenting in two generations: looking backwards and looking forwards. In: Madge N, ed. *Families at risk.* London: Heinemann Educational, 1983;**10**:60–98.
11 Brown GW, Rutter M. The measurement of family activities and relationships: a methological study. *Human Relations* 1966;**19**:241–63.
12 Crowell JA, Feldman SS. Mothers' internal models of relationship and children's behavioural and developmental status: a study of mother–child interaction. *Child Dev* 1988;**59**:1273–85.
13 Protchasha J, Di Clemente D. Towards a comprehensive model of change in treating addictive behaviour: processes of change. In: Miller R, Heather N, eds. *Treating addictive behaviour.* London: Plenum Press, 1986:3–27.

14 Bentovim A, Elton A, Tranter M. Prognosis for rehabilitation after abuse. *Adoption and Fostering* 1987;**11**:26–31.
15 Jones D. The untreatable family. *Child Abuse Negl* 1987;**11**:109–20.
16 Gent M. The 'parent–child game': an innovative approach to parenting assessment and training with relevance to child abuse. *Nursing Standard* 1991;5, **45**:16–7.
17 Dunn J, Kendrick C. Temperamental differences, family relationships and young children's response to change within the family. *Ciba Foundation symposium 89: temperamental differences in infants and young children.* London: Pitman, 1982:87–105.
18 Familaro D, Kinsaharff R, Bunschoft D, Spvah T, Benton A. Parental compliance to court order treatment interventions in cases of child maltreatment. *Child Abuse Negl* 1989;**13**:507–11.
19 Wolfe D, Aragona J, Kandman J, Sandler J. The importance of adjudication in the treatment of child abusers. *Child Abuse Negl* 1980;**4**:127–75.
20 Black D, Wolkind S, Harris Hendricks J, eds. *Child psychiatry and the law.* London: Gaskell and Royal College of Psychiatrists, 1989.

Further reading

Rutter M. *Maternal deprivation reassessed.* 2nd Ed. Harmondsworth: Penguin, 1983.
Goldstein J, Freud AJ. *Beyond the best interest of the child.* London: Barnett Books, 1980.
Adcock M, White R, eds. *Good enough parenting: a framework for assessment.* London: British Agencies for Adoption and Fostering, 1985.

12. Treatment of delinquents

Carol Sheldrick

Definition

As West points out, delinquency is a sociolegal category.[1] The definition of a juvenile delinquent, in the UK at least, is a young person between the age of 10 (the age of "criminal responsibility") and 17 years who has been prosecuted and found guilty of an offence that would be classified as a "crime" if committed by an adult. These offences normally result in the opening of a criminal record file at Scotland Yard but do not include more minor drunk and disorderly, common assault, and motoring offences.

The size of the problem

Research findings are consistent in showing that most young people (particularly boys) have committed delinquent acts at some time. Not all boys appear in court, but self report studies do pick out many of the boys with official records, and the higher the score on a schedule of self reported offences the greater the likelihood of the young person having an official conviction record.[2-4] Farrington,[5] using data from the Cambridge study, a longitudinal study of 400 boys living in inner London and selected randomly from six adjacent primary schools,[4 6-8] showed that up to the age of 32, over one third were convicted of criminal offences. The peak age for the number of offenders and the number of offences was 17, but roughly equal numbers of offences were committed by males as juveniles (age 10–16), as young adults (age 17–20), and as adults (21–32). The men who were first convicted at the earliest ages tended to become the most persistent offenders and committed large numbers of offences at high rates over long time periods. Despite this, earlier work by West, showed that only about one quarter of adolescent offenders continued to offend into their twenties.[7]

Much less research has been carried out on females but figures quoted by Farrington suggested that the ratio of males to females acquiring a criminal record was about 3·5–4·5:1.[9]

Implications for management

It is clear from this research that a certain amount of law breaking is the norm, particularly for males, and does not necessarily imply any appreciable degree of personal maladjustment. Many youths only appear in court once and only a small proportion show a persistent pattern of delinquency. Though it may seem appropriate to intervene as early as possible in the lives of delinquents, research suggests otherwise.

The dangers of intervention

The judicial process

There are differing theories about the judicial response to delinquency. The work of Farrington *et al* has shown that the first appearance in court tends to be followed by an increase in delinquent activities as well as increases in hostile attitudes towards the police and aggressive attitudes and behaviour.[10] This study suggests that a first court appearance (and public labelling) has a deleterious effect, and probably more so if the consequences are trivial. A study by McCord, however, suggests otherwise.[11]

In Britain we lock up a higher proportion of our population than most other Western European countries. At one time it was hoped that institutional treatments would be therapeutic and reformative in their effects. Unfortunately this has not proved to be so and some studies from America show that non-custodial approaches do better than institutional ones.[12 13] McCord, in the study referred to above, showed that incarcerated boys do not do better with respect to recidivism than those receiving more lenient sentences.[11] In England there is no evidence that the borstal (now renamed the young offender) system is effective in influencing long term recidivism. Sixty four per cent of trainees released in 1972 were reconvicted within two years; the figure for boys under the age of 17 years was even higher, at 79%.[14]

It seems unlikely that institutional treatment, retraining, and punishment are effective in decreasing delinquency. It is even possible that there is a harmful effect because of the alienation, stigmatisation, and "contamination" suffered by those who are incarcerated with other offenders.

Community based programmes

Better results would have been anticipated from community based, non-punitive programmes. Unfortunately this has not been borne out by the evidence. One study by O'Donnell *et al* was of young people referred for behavioural problems to a contingency behavioural management programme by schools and also by the police, courts, and social welfare agencies.[15] Youths were randomly assigned to a treatment group or a non-treatment control group. Non-delinquent youths in the treatment group were found to be more likely to offend than those placed in the non-treatment control group, particularly if they had been in treatment for more than one year. The only explanation that seemed plausible was that, through the group meetings and shared activities organised by the professionals, those with no previous arrests established friendships with young people who had committed offences. An important study by McCord looked at boys aged 5–13 years who were thought to be at risk of developing delinquency, but who had not yet done so.[16] It noted the long term effects of a treatment programme for boys and their families based on a 30 year follow up of over 500 men, one half of whom had been randomly assigned to a treatment programme for an average of five years. Treatment consisted of counselling for the boy and his family, introduction to community programmes and summer camps, provision of medical and psychiatric assistance, as well as tutoring in academic subjects. The treated group actually fared worse than the control group on such measures as criminal behaviour, death at a young age, stress related disease, alcoholism, serious mental illness, occupational status, and job satisfaction. The author does not give an explanation for the findings. It is possible that the professional input gave the boys and their families unrealistic expectations about the future that could not be fulfilled, that the professional input "labelled" the families and undermined their ability to develop their own strategies and networks for coping with problems, or that the input offered was not sufficiently problem-orientated and focused.

More successful community based programmes have been developed, however, mostly in North America, and reviewed by Stumphauzer.[17]

Attempts at diversion

The courts

It is clear from this research that the diversion of young people from certain interventions, particularly those of the courts and the prison system, is desirable.

In Britain the Children and Young Persons Act 1969 was introduced to prevent children coming to court for criminal proceedings.[18] Before 1971 children could be given a warning if apprehended while committing an offence. This was an informal procedure, conducted at the discretion of the police officer and not recorded officially. The 1969 act gave statutory sanction for police cautioning as a means of diverting children from the courts. The caution is usually administered, with the consent of the child, parents, and victim, in a formal way to emphasise the gravity of the situation. Sometimes the police undertake follow up supervision and guidance, or they may refer the child to the social service department on a voluntary basis.

In 1979, the year when the legislation was fully implemented, it was found that cautioning increased,[19] which led Farrington and Bennett to believe that this had produced a widening of the net, so that official cautions had tended to replace informal, unrecorded warnings rather than being used in place of court appearances.[20]

Since then, however, the situation appears to have changed for the better. Richardson and Tutt,[21] using data from the Home Office,[22] pointed out that there was a 23·2% decrease in the number of 10–16 year olds in the population in England and Wales over the 10 years 1979–88. Over 55% fewer juveniles, however, entered the formal court system during 1988 than did in 1979, a very dramatic diversion of young people away from the courts.

In Scotland the police do not make the decisions as to when a young person should be cautioned, referred to a social agency, or passed on to a magistrates court. A reporter is an official who sifts complaints from the police and others and decides which cases can be dealt with informally and which cases need to be passed on for a formal tribunal hearing. Unlike courts, the hearings have no power to impose fines or make committals to penal institutions. Only on instructions from the Lord Advocate are a small number of children prosecuted in the Sheriff Court or High Court, usually for serious offences against the person.

The use of courts for care proceedings and intervention in the community

In England courts have basically two types of case to hear: care proceedings and criminal proceedings. Under the age of 10 years a child cannot be found guilty of a crime (except homicide) and between 10 and 14 years should not be prosecuted for a crime. This means that all those under the age of 14 years should come before the courts for care proceedings only. An additional safeguard is that the Children and Young Persons Act 1969,[18] replaced by the Children Act 1989,[23] sets out criteria for taking out care proceedings. Under the terms of the Children Act 1989, a care order may no longer be imposed as a sentence in criminal proceedings. However the fact that a child has committed an offence may indicate that he or she is suffering, or likely to suffer, significant harm, so that the local authority may apply for a care order in respect of that child.

The use of supervision orders

These orders were originally introduced in the act of 1969[18] as a means of dealing with offenders through an intermediate treatment programme (see below). They can now be linked to a number of disposals (Children Act 1989[23] and Criminal Justice Act 1982[24]). Supervision orders may still be made in criminal proceedings, the statutory responsibility lying with the local social services or, in the case of older juveniles, with the probation service. The primary consideration is to "advise, assist and befriend" and not to protect the public, though the supervisor can return the young person to court if the terms of the order are breached.

Supervision orders with a supervised activity requirement

The supervised activity requirement can be made by magistrates, and social services have to accept it. Placements are usually drawn from the intermediate treatment scheme.

Intermediate treatment has been adopted since the white paper *Children in Trouble* was published by the Home Office.[25] The aim is to fill the gap between simple supervision and removal from home. It is designed to allow the child to remain in his home, but bring him into contact with a different environment, interests, and experiences that may be beneficial to him and enable him to share them with other children who have not been before the courts. Although intermediate treatment is usually community based, it can be provided in a residential facility for up to 90 days. As Cawson points out, the end of the 1970s saw two major developments in practice: "intensive intermediate treatment" to provide a real alternative to removal from home, and the introduction of new methods for working with groups.[26] Nevertheless there is still substantial disagreement within social work as to the desirability of programmes that are an alternative to custody, and many intermediate treatment programmes are still focused on non-offenders, or even exclude serious delinquents.

Custodial sentencing

In Britain we have a history of locking up large numbers of young people. The numbers dealt with in this way escalated dramatically during the 1960s and 1970s,[27] and particularly so immediately after the introduction of the Criminal Justice Act 1982.[28] These trends were seen for girls as well as boys.

The situation during the 1980s, however, changed for the better. As has already been noted, there has been a large increase in the numbers of young people diverted from the courts in Britain during 1979–89. The same trend has been mirrored by the numbers of young people receiving custodial sentences—that is, 7097 in 1979 and 2176 in 1988.[22]

It is of interest to note that similar changes have occurred within the child care system, a great increase in the provision of secure accommodation having occurred in the 1970s, with a decline in its provision during the past decade.[29]

Is treatment of delinquency possible?

Causes of offending

Numerous studies have shown that delinquency tends to be much more common in adolescents coming from certain kinds of family and social backgrounds. The most important variables associated with juvenile delinquency are: large family size, poverty, parental criminality, marital conflict, poor parental supervision, cruel, passive, or neglecting attitudes, and erratic or harsh discipline.[4 30 31] Farrington has shown that the childhood predictors of conviction up to the age of 32 can be grouped into six major conceptual categories: socioeconomic deprivation, poor parental child rearing, family deviance, school problems, hyperactivity-impulsivity-attention deficit, and antisocial child behaviour. He suggests that the link between antisocial child behaviour[5] and offending probably reflects an underlying construct of antisocial personality, and goes on to suggest that the other five constructs are possible causes of offending.

Implications for treatment

The implications for planning treatment from these considerations are considerable. Whatever the theoretical starting point it is

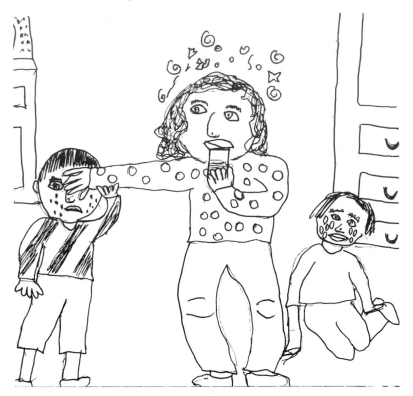

Harsh and neglectful parenting can be linked with delinquency in the child

generally agreed that there is no single cause of delinquency; the factors initiating delinquency are probably not the same as those maintaining it. It is not clear how the various factors interact, and most of those identified tend to be interrelated anyway. As discussed by Rutter and Giller, it is difficult to know which possible cause to treat, particularly bearing in mind the gap between identifying a damaging influence and knowing how to mitigate or eliminate it.[32]

The work of Farrington suggests that potential offenders can be identified at an early age with a reasonable degree of accuracy and that, on the basis of current empirical evidence, the most helpful methods of reducing juvenile offending are through parental training and educational programmes.[5] Other possible interventions include giving more economic resources to poor families, providing juveniles with socially approved opportunities for excitement and risk taking, deterring offending through an increased probability and level of penalty (although this also has dangers), increasing the physical security or surveillance of potential targets, and encouraging resistance to antisocial peer pressures.

Who to target?

The individual and the family

A medical model of delinquency has been in vogue for many years. Within this model the major determinants of delinquent behaviour are regarded as being located within the individual, the maladjusted personality being the result of genetic inheritance or the product of early experiences and relationships, especially from within the family.[33] Though such a model might suggest a psychotherapeutic approach to the treatment of delinquents, psychotherapy has been found to be of value with only a relatively small number of anxious, introverted young people who are aware of their personal problems and who want help for them. In the past 20 years there has been a considerable increase in the application of behavioural treatment programmes for antisocial and aggressive behaviour. Yule has reviewed the most important of these techniques.[34]

The most extensive behavioural family intervention studies have been those undertaken by Patterson and his colleagues at the Oregon social learning centre.[35 37] Both aggressive children and delinquents have been treated using a behaviourally oriented parent training programme. Parents are helped to use positive, non-coercive methods of control; to interact more positively as a family; to monitor their children's activities better and to deal more decisively with deviant behaviour; to negotiate behavioural contracts with their children; and to develop improved social problem solving skills. The findings have shown that both aggression and stealing can be noticeably reduced by this approach, but that the benefits are much shorter lived with young people who steal. Though this approach offers great promise, the studies published so far have been flawed by methodological difficulties. Kazdin et al are researching further the possible benefits of parent management training and cognitive-behavioural problem solving skills (see also chapter 4 in this book).[38 39]

An important development has been the establishment of residential group homes, closely integrated with the community and run on behavioural lines. The best example of this approach is provided by the achievement place studies.[40-44] The model provides a community based, family style, group home treatment programme for six to eight youths aged 12–15 years who are in danger of being institutionalised. The programme is administered by a couple referred to as teaching parents, who have had a year's professional training. The goal of the programme is to establish through reinforcement, modelling, and instruction the skills needed in the social, self care, academic, and prevocational areas that the youths have not acquired. There appears to be an appreciable reduction in offending during treatment, but no advantages at one year follow up.[45]

As Farrington postulates, if low intelligence and school problems are causes of offending then any programme that leads to an increase in school success should lead to a decrease in offending.[5] He quotes the Perry preschool project carried out in Michigan by Schweinhart and Weikart.[46] This "Head Start" programme and a later follow up study of this group by Berrueta-Clement et al[47] suggest great promise, but the study requires replication (see also chapter 14).

The residential establishment

Delinquent children who repeatedly come to the attention of the authorities tend, in this country at least, to end up in some form of residential care, and much Home Office research has been directed towards evaluating and comparing such institutions.

Cross institutional designs have been used to look at the large differences that exist between institutions in the behaviour shown by similar types of residents while they are in their care. The first Home Office cross institutional study was designed and carried out by Sinclair.[48 49] The study was concerned to examine the probation hostel system, where it was found that the proportions of boys leaving the hostels prematurely as a result of absconding or further offending ranged from 14% to 78%. Sinclair found that certain qualities of the staff, in particular the wardens, were important. By using the Jesness staff attitudes questionnaires it was found that wardens with the lowest rate of premature leaving were those who ran a strictly disciplined hostel, but who also expressed warmth towards the boys and were in agreement with their wives about how the hostel should be run.[50] Those who were harsh, emotionally distant, lax, permissive, or who disagreed with their wives about hostel policy tended to have high drop-out rates from their hostels.

Many young people are placed in community homes with education on the premises (CH(E)s). (Before the Children and Young Persons Act 1969[18] these were known as approved schools.) Studies by Millham et al[51] and Sinclair and Clarke[52] have shown that successful schools are dependent on qualities of staff and combine a harmonious atmosphere, good staff–pupil relationships, kindness, consistency, firmness, with high expectations, a high level of activities, and vocational training. Dunlop's more detailed study of eight CH(E)s, catering for boys aged 13–15 on admission, showed that schools that appeared to lay emphasis on trade training and on mature and responsible behaviour had lower rates of both absconding and other forms of misbehaviour during attendance as well as having marginally, though appreciably, lower reconviction rates.[53]

In their comparison of 12 inner London secondary schools, Rutter et al showed that delinquency rates were probably affected by school factors such as appropriately high expectations, good group management, effective feedback to the children with ample use of praise, the setting of good models of behaviour by teachers, pleasant working conditions, and giving pupils positions of trust and responsibility.[54]

The therapist

Research into institutions and the use of specific techniques has led to an increasing awareness of the importance of therapist qualities. As early as 1967, Truax and Carkhuff's work with adults being treated with Rogerian counselling emphasised that effective counsellors were characterised by genuineness, empathy, and non-possessive warmth.[55] Subsequent work has shown a great deal of inconsistency in the effects of these therapist variables,[56] and other studies have suggested that different qualities are important. Alexander et al examined therapist variables in relation to interventions with families of delinquents.[57] They found that 60% of the outcome variance in treated cases was accounted for by structuring and relationship skills (relationship skills being composed of several behaviourally defined categories including affection, warmth, and humour) (see also the section on therapist variables in chapter 4 by McAuley in this book). Kolvin et al found substantial differences between therapists in their effectiveness in treating children, but that the important qualities were extroversion, assertiveness, and openness.[58] Clearly, research indicates that therapist qualities are important, but further studies are required to establish which are the most important ones and whether or not they can be taught.

Is there a medical role in the treatment of delinquency?

Assessment of delinquents

Though delinquents have many features in common, it has often been observed that some patterns of delinquency overlap with aggression, emotional disturbance, poor peer relationships, hyperactivity, and attentional deficits. These problems may well require assessment and treatment in their own right, which can best be provided by a multidisciplinary team based in a child psychiatry department or child guidance clinic. These teams are usually headed by a medically qualified practitioner, but the medical role in the assessment and treatment of delinquency is probably a limited one.

Counselling and psychotherapy, based on the establishment of a personal relationship, have rarely proved successful except—as already noted—for a small minority of rather anxious, introverted young people who are aware of their personal problems and want help with them. Overt neurological disorder or severe psychiatric abnormality are met with only occasionally in adolescent offenders. Those with hyperactivity and attentional deficits may benefit from medication, and those with emotional disturbance may benefit from individual or family psychotherapy. However, the numbers that can be helped in these ways are few. For the majority, treatment aims are probably best directed towards improving the educational, vocational, practical, and social skills of the individual; and a problem oriented approach to assessment and treatment of young offenders promises to be the most effective. Such an approach has been described by Stumphauzer.[17]

Requests for psychiatric court reports

Despite the fact that the medical role in the assessment and treatment of delinquency is limited, psychiatrists are often asked to prepare reports on young offenders for the court. There are a number of different issues on which they are asked to advise. The first, and most obvious, is to comment on the presence (or absence) of mental illness. Signs that might suggest this are reports of self damage, extreme changes of mood, and recent changes in personality. A history of solvent or drug abuse may also give cause for

> ## Box 1—Indications for psychiatric interventions or court involvement in delinquency
>
> When delinquency is part of:
> - An anxious introverted personality
> - Hyperkinesis or attention deficit disorder
> - Self damage, extreme changes of mood, recent changes in personality
> - Solvent or drug abuse
> - Developmental delays or associated physical illness (ie, speech disorders, enuresis, epilepsy)
> - Bizarre or unusual behaviour
> - Past or family history of psychiatric illness or intervention
> - Intact families with dysfunctional patterns of interaction
> - Dangerous behaviour such as sexual deviancy, fire setting, serious assaults against others.

concern. Aspects of the background history, in the absence of any obvious symptoms, such as a history of mental illness in the family, may also lead to the request for a psychiatric opinion. A psychiatrist may also be involved in the assessment and management of some developmental delays, physical conditions, and illnesses, especially if there is an emotional component. The investigations for speech disorder, enuresis, and epilepsy provide examples: the hyperkinetic syndrome of childhood deserves special investigation and treatment. A request may be made for an adolescent to be seen alone, or with his family, and in this context it may be possible for a psychiatrist to express a view on the personality and emotional development of the young person, other members of the family, or on the functioning of the family as a whole.

Other indications for assessment are unusual or bizarre behaviour either reported in the past, possibly at the time of an offence, or even witnessed in court during a hearing. Inexplicable, repetitive offending, sexual deviancy, and dangerous behaviour, such as fire setting and serious assault against another person, may lead to a psychiatric referral.

As with adults, a specific request for assessment of dangerousness, fitness to plead, diminished responsibility, and treatability within the resources of the health service may be requested of psychiatrists. In addition they are often asked to advise on, or support recommendations for, placements within the child care system, and often have an important role in consulting to establishments within that system.

Box 2—Strategies in forensic adolescent psychiatry

Problem oriented approach to assessment and treatment

Improving educational, vocational, practical, and social skills of individuals

Warmth, consistency, firmness, high but appropriate expectations, definition of objectives

Court reports for assessment of:
- Dangerousness
- Fitness to plead
- Diminished responsibility
- Treatability within the resources of the NHS
- Recommendations for placements within the child care system.

Conclusion

The medical role in the treatment of delinquency is a limited one. There is conflicting evidence as to whether treatment aims should be directed towards the individual, to the family, the institution, or the therapist. Nevertheless, there seems to be a consensus of opinion that short term, focused therapies aimed at improving educational, vocational, and social skills, possibly from a preschool age, are the most effective. Any treatment gains achieved while in residential care appear to be short lived. It therefore seems that this should be reserved for those individuals who commit repeated, violent crimes and for those from very damaging family backgrounds who repeatedly abscond or absent themselves from community based programmes.

1 West DJ. Delinquency. In: Rutter M, Hersov L, eds. *Child psychiatry: modern approaches*. Oxford: Blackwell Scientific Publications, 1985:414–23.
2 Belson WA. *Juvenile theft: the causal factors*. London: Harper and Row, 1975.
3 Hardt RH, Hardt SP. On determining the quality of the delinquency self-report method. *Journal of Research in Crime and Delinquency* 1977;**14**:247–61.
4 West DJ, Farrington DP. *Who becomes delinquent?* London: Heinemann Educational Books, 1973.
5 Farrington DP. Implications of criminal career research for the prevention of offending. *J Adolesc* 1990;**13**:93–113.
6 West DJ. *Present conduct and future delinqucy*. London: Heinemann Educational Books, 1969.
7 West DJ. *Delinquency: its roots, careers and prospects*. London: Heinemann Educational Books, 1982.
8 West DJ, Farrington DP. *The delinquent way of life*. London: Heinemann Educational Books, 1977.
9 Farrington DP. The prevalence of convictions. *British Journal of Criminology* 1981;**21**:173–5.
10 Farrington DP, Osborn SG, West DJ. The persistence of labelling effects. *British Journal of Criminology* 1978;**18**:277–84.
11 McCord J. Deterrence and the light touch of the law. In: Farrington DP,

Gunn J, eds. *Reactions of crime: the police, courts, and prisons*. Chichester: John Wiley, 1985:73–85.

12 Empey LT, Erickson ML. *The provo experiment: evaluating community control of delinquency*. Lexington, Massachusetts: D C Heath, 1972.

13 Wright WE, Dixon MC. Community prevention and treatment of juvenile delinquency: a review of evaluation studies. *Journal of Research in Crime and Delinquency* 1977;14:35–67.

14 Home Office. *Report on the work of the prison department*. London: HMSO, 1975. (Cmnd 6542.)

15 O'Donnell CR, Lydgate T, Fo WSO. The buddy system: review and follow-up. *Child Behaviour Therapy* 1979;1:161–9.

16 McCord J. A thirty year follow-up of treatment effects. *Am Psychol* 1978;33:284–9.

17 Stumphauzer JS. *Helping delinquents change: a treatment manual of social learning approaches*. New York: The Haworth Press, 1986.

18 Home Office. *Children and young persons act*. London: HMSO, 1969:ch 54.

19 Home Office. *Criminal statistics England and Wales, 1978*. London: HMSO, 1979.

20 Farrington DP, Bennett T. Police cautioning of juveniles in London. *British Journal of Criminology* 1981;21:277–84.

21 Richardson N, Tutt N. Delinquency and social policy 1979–1989. *Association of Child Psychology and Psychiatry Newsletter* 1991;13(1):4–9.

22 Home Office. *Criminal statistics England and Wales, 1988*. London: HMSO, 1989.

23 Department of Health. *Children act*. London: HMSO, 1989:ch 41.

24 Home Office. *Criminal justice act 1982*. London: HMSO, 1982:ch 48.

25 Home Office. *Children in trouble*. London: HMSO, 1968. (Cmnd 3601).

26 Cawson P. Intermediate treatment. *J Child Psychol Psychiatry* 1985;26:675–81.

27 Rutherford A. Why should courts make non-custodial orders? *Juvenile offenders: care, control or custody*. Howard League Day Conference Report, London, 1980.

28 Home Office. *Criminal justice act 1982: reception into prison department establishments of young offenders*. London: HMSO, 1984.

29 Cawson P. *Long term secure accommodation: a review of evidence and discussion of London's needs*. London: London Borough's Children's Regional Planning Committee, 1986.

30 McCord J. Some child-rearing antecedents of criminal behaviour in adult men. *J Pers Soc Psychol* 1979;37:1477–6.

31 Wadsworth M. *Roots of delinquency: infancy, adolescence and crime*. Oxford: Martin Robertson, 1979.

32 Rutter M, Giller H. *Juvenile delinquency: trends and perspectives*. Harmondsworth: Penguin Books, 1983.

33 Bowlby J. *Forty-four juvenile thieves*. London: Baillière, Tindall and Cox, 1946.

34 Yule W. Behavioural approaches. In: Rutter M, Hersov L, eds. *Child and adolescent psychiatry: modern approaches*. Oxford: Blackwell Scientific Publications, 1985:794–808.

35 Patterson GR, Cobb JA, Ray RS. A social engineering technology for retraining the families of aggressive boys. In: Adams HE, Unikel IP, eds. *Issues and trends in behaviour therapy*. Springfield, Illinois: Charles C Thomas, 1973:139–210.

36 Patterson GR. Interventions for boys with conduct problems: multiple settings, treatments and criteria. *J Consult Clin Psychol* 1974;43:471–81.

37 Patterson GR. Treatment for children with conduct problems: a review of outcome studies. In: Feshbach S, Fraczek A, eds. *Aggression and behaviour change: biological and social processes*. New York: Praeger, 1979:83–138.

38 Kazdin AE, Esveldt-Dawson K, French NH, Unis AS. Effects of parent

165

management training and problem-solving skills training in the treatment of antisocial child behaviour. *J Am Acad Child Adolesc Psychiatr* 1987;**26**:416–24.

39 Kazdin AE. Premature termination from treatment among children referred for antisocial behaviour. *J Child Psychol Psychiatry* 1990;**31**:415–25.

40 Fixsen DL, Phillips EL, Wolf MM. Achievement place: experiments in self government with predelinquents. *J Appl Behav Anal* 1973;**6**:31–49.

41 Hoefler SA, Bornstein PH. Achievement place: an evaluative review. *Crim Justice and Behaviour* 1975;**2**:146–68.

42 Phillips EL. Achievement place: token reinforcement procedures in a home-style rehabilitation setting for predelinquent boys. *J Appl Behav Anal* 1968;**1**:213–23.

43 Phillips EL, Phillips EA, Fixsen DL, Wolf MM. Achievement place: modification of the behaviours of predelinquent boys within a company economy. *J Appl Behav Anal* 1971;**4**:45–59.

44 Phillips EL, Phillips EA, Fixsen DL, Wolf MM. Achievement place: behaviour shaping works for delinquents. *Psychology Today* 1973:June 75–9.

45 Kirigen KA, Braukmann CJ, Atwater JD, Wolf MM. An evaluation of teaching family (achievement place) group homes for juvenile offenders. *J Appl Behav Anal* 1982;**15**:1–16.

46 Schweinhart LJ, Weikart DP. *Young children grow up*. Ypsilanti, Michigan: High/Scope, 1980.

47 Berrueta-Clement JR, Schweinhart LJ, Barnett WS, Epstein AS, Weikart DP. *Changed lives*. Ypsilanti, Michigan: High/Scope, 1984.

48 Sinclair IAC. *Hostel for probationers*. Home Office Research Study No 6. London: HMSO, 1971.

49 Sinclair IAC. The influence of wardens and matrons on probation hostels: a study of quasi-family institution. In: Tizard J, Sinclair IAC, Clarke RVG, eds. *Varieties of residential experience*. London: Routledge and Kegan Paul, 1975:122–40.

50 Jesness CF. *The Fricot ranch study*. Research report No 47. Sacramento: California Department of Youth Study, 1965.

51 Millham S, Bullock R, Cherret P. *After grace—teeth: a comparative study of the residential experiences of boys in approved schools*. London: Human Context Books, 1975.

52 Sinclair IAC, Clarke RVG. Predicting, treating and explaining delinquency: the lessons from research on institutions. In: Feldman P, ed. *Developments in the study of criminal behaviour. Vol I. The prevention and control of offending*. Chichester: John Wiley, 1982:51–78.

53 Dunlop AB. *The approved school experience*. Home Office research study No 25. London: HMSO, 1974.

54 Rutter M, Maughan B, Mortimer P, Ousten J, Smith A. Fifteen thousand hours: secondary schools and their effects on children. London: Open Books, 1979.

55 Truax CB, Carkhuff RR. *Towards effective counselling and psychotherapy: training and practice*. Chicago: Aldin, 1967.

56 Mitchell KM, Bozarth JD, Krauft CC. A reappraisal of the therapeutic effectiveness of accurate empathy, non-possessive warmth and genuiness. In: Gurman AS, Razin AM, eds. *Effective psychotherapy: a handbook of research*. New York: Pergamon Press, 1977:482–502.

57 Alexander JF, Barton C, Schiavo RS, Parsons BV. Systems-behavioural intervention with families of delinquents: therapist characteristics, family behaviour and outcome. *J Consult Clin Psychol* 1976;**44**:656–64.

58 Kolvin I, Garside RF, Nicol AR, MacMillan A, Wolstenholme F, Leitch IM. *Help starts here: the maladjusted child in the ordinary school*. London: Tavistock, 1981.

13. Psychiatric treatment for children—the organisation of services

Fiona Subostky

The Court report in 1976 laid down the classic blueprint for the organisation of children's mental health services.[1] Since then the priorities of health and other services have changed.[2] Social services in some parts of the country have had to redirect social workers from child guidance to child protection work, often because of the major increase in reporting of child sexual abuse, and now also have to consider the implications of the Children Act 1989.[3] Education services have had two major education acts to deal with,[4,5] and they are subject to the turbulence of further continued reform.

This chapter looks at dynamics more than structures and offers observations on how modern approaches, especially of health economics, are shaping an inner London child psychiatry service in the new context of the NHS reforms.[6]

Methodologies to improve services

MARGINAL COST BENEFIT ANALYSIS

Marginal analysis in health economics is a method of evaluation when planning a service programme to find the most cost beneficial way of proceeding.[7] The approach of marginal analysis:

(a) Acknowledges the limitations of resources. The child psychiatry service probably has a fixed budget, and opportunities for increased funding look limited.

(b) Proceeds from current available provision and use of resources. The first step in planning is not therefore to survey the hypothetical "child psychiatric needs" of the whole population and from this recommend "ideal provision", but to look at current provision, its uptake, and effectiveness.

(c) Tries to establish priorities for a given type of provision, rather than to set an arbitrary standard. It seems difficult in the usual multidisciplinary child psychiatry setting for instance, to answer the question "which cases would not benefit from long term child psychotherapy?". On the other hand, a "marginal" type of question—"What sort of cases have in the last year benefited least from long term individual psychotherapy?" has been found to be more readily answerable, and provides an opportunity for the future more effective direction of resources.

(d) Tries to identify the range of costs, both for the service and its users. These could include (for the child and his or her family attending child psychiatry outpatient appointments) for example, costs of distress, stigmatisation, loss of education and income, and disruption of household arrangements. For the child psychiatry service costs could include resources devoted to the treatment, the stressfulness of the case, and the opportunity cost of not offering the resource to another, more responsive, case.

(e) Tries to identify the range of benefits—for instance, acceptability, availability, efficacy of treatment, accessibility, and equitability. In child psychiatry the child whose symptoms are relieved is not the only beneficiary; there are gains for the parents and siblings, and often also the school. "Benefits" for the service could include contributing to the fulfilment of the service contract, the opportunity for learning and research, and variety.

(f) Concentrates on marginal rather than average costs and benefits. So far, costings in child psychiatry are very rudimentary, because of the non-standard nature of problems, situations, and interventions. However, it is clear that it would be cheaper (and easier) for an established programme—say of group work for sexually abused children—to take on a few extra cases, than it would be to provide a new, similar programme for a small number of children not far away. This is even more obvious for expensive provision such as adolescent inpatient admissions.

(g) Establishes a framework in which judgments of relative benefit are made explicit and thus trade offs are clearer. Formal measurement of costs and benefits is limited and difficult in child psychiatry. Informally, however, extreme categorisations of the ratios of cost to benefit of cases have been found acceptable and are the subject of further study. For instance, most clinicians, when asked, could respond to the question "Which of your recent cases represented the poorest clinical gain in relation to the resources put in?". Then, if such cases have common characteristics, there is the possibility of considering limiting input at an earlier stage, in order to devote resources elsewhere.

AUDIT

For child psychiatry, audit offers a way of improving treatments and services using local data and nationally available information educationally, even when the resources and opportunities for mounting double blind controlled trials are not available.

In our district, multidisciplinary audit in child psychiatry is being used explicitly to improve the service offered at a number of levels as recommended by the Royal College of Psychiatrists.[8]

Team level

Quality of case notes—extremely simple standards have been found to be robust but revealing:

- Can the file be found?
- Is the cover/front sheet information complete?
- Are the notes filed correctly?
- Is there a typed first assessment?
- Have the general practitioner (GP) and referrer been informed of the outcome of assessment?
- Is there a note of action in the last six months, or a letter to GP and referrer advising of closure?

After 15 months, standards have considerably improved.

Commissioners' requirements—This year, 1993; the commissioners asked for the following to be audited:

- After a GP referral, in 80% of cases a meaningful reply should be sent to the patients/clients within two weeks,
- Time for response to GP after first assessment to be reported,
- Waiting time for appointment.

Auditing these has also led to an improvement in standards, although more administrative support and appropriate computerised information systems are necessary for full implementation.

Interteam level

The four consultant teams of the district hold audit meetings each term, with an educational focus on topics of major treatment relevance, to consider current practice and "best practice" advice and how to modify management in the light of this. "Soiling" and "hyperactivity/conduct disorder" have been considered so far.

Planning group level

At the district planning group level audit relevant to service is coordinated by means of:

- General information review,
- Promotion of specific audit projects,
- Organisation of other quality oriented projects such as patient satisfaction surveys, etc,
- Resource issues review,
- Coordination of other audit results for annual review and report to commissioners,
- Liaison with other audit committees within the hospital and at regional level.

OUTCOME MEASURES

Outcome studies of treatment in child psychiatry are being performed more often now and are encouraging,[9–11] but outcome measures suitable for general use are not yet available. This is not surprising given the variety of contributory factors to childhood mental disorder, the degree of comorbidity, and the eclecticism of interventions. As databases become more widespread, however, it is worthwhile beginning with what seems feasible locally.

Administrative outcomes

Administrative outcomes are the simplest to measure, and are worth monitoring—for example:

- Referral not accepted,
- Referral withdrawn,
- Case attended,
- Case never attended.

Referrals have been monitored on this basis at local clinics for several years, so comparisons and trends are apparent. Other clinics have found useful slightly more complicated categorisations, adding in mode of discharge.[12 13]

Therapeutic outcome measures

Systematic attempts to measure therapeutic outcome are now being evaluated.[9] What should be done with outcome measure results? At present, differences between different centres for apparently the same condition would be very difficult to evaluate, but within the same centre outcomes should be an aid to decision making. Repeated measures of progress on individual cases would also be a guide to when intervention could be terminated.

In the future, quality adjusted life year (QALY) type measures may be evaluated,[14] to answer not only "within programme" but "between programme" questions—such as, What are the comparative costs and therapeutic gains of an average child psychiatry and an average paediatric course of treatment?

Performance indicators

The national requirements of the Körner report are ill suited to child psychiatry,[15] but are still collected through most hospitals' patient administration systems. A survey of all consultant child psychiatrists in the region, which I conducted, showed that each Körner information requirement was interpreted variously. As a result of attempts to increase local validity (meaningfulness), central reliability was completely lost. However, as Jenkins has rightly pointed out, process measures such as these should not be used as a proxy for outcome measures.[16]

Health outcomes

The monitoring of childhood "health states" such as the para-suicide and suicide rates, the incidence of psychiatric disturbance, and the emotional impact of psychosocial disadvantage, has been recommended as an appropriate method of measuring outcome for child psychiatry.[16] This appears bizarre to the clinician—rather like judging the performance of the accident and emergency consultant by the number of road accidents, and shows how important it is to have agreed objectives for a service before setting out to measure its effectiveness. However, population morbidity measures (such as the child abuse rate) could certainly help to indicate priorities for intervention.

CONSUMER RESEARCH AND QUALITY

"Consumerist" approaches are now important in evaluating, and therefore determining, services. Who is the consumer in child psychiatry?

The child and the family

Preparatory information—A local survey[17] supported other findings[18 19] that parental understanding of child psychiatry services is limited. As outcomes may be better if expectations of family and clinic are congruent,[20] we have reviewed information sent out at the different clinics and are in the process of improving it.

Improving attendance rate—Non-attendance at appointments is commonly noted in child psychiatry,[13] and can be a considerable waste of professional time. Implementing the suggestion to telephone some families beforehand has helped reduce the non-attendance rate in one of the local teams.[21 22] Requiring questionnaire completion was thought to be too demanding for our population,[22 23] as even routine confirmation of appointment is only erratically complied with.

Waiting time—A local survey showed that parents who thought the wait for appointment was "too long" had waited an average of 8·6 weeks; parents who thought the wait was "OK" had waited a mean of 7·1 weeks,[17] Efforts are made to keep the waiting time down to six weeks if possible. If, as has sometimes happened because of staff cuts, a waiting list of three months develops at a clinic then referrers are advised about alternatives.

Although a longer waiting time for an appointment has been seen to reduce the likelihood of attendance,[24] audit of one local team's attendance rate showed a surprising tendency for offer of a rapid appointment (within 1–3 weeks) to be associated with a higher failure rate, so that time taken over checking willingness to attend was concluded to be more important.

Patient satisfaction: process—Satisfaction with "process" variables—such as ease of finding the department, the pleasantness of the waiting area, the acceptability of the toys and reading material—is currently being surveyed in our hospital department. It is hoped that this will disclose opportunities for improvement, and also possibly provide ways of comparing different sites in a standardised way, and where necessary underpin arguments for upgrading of facilities.

Patient satisfaction: outcome—Successful attempts to measure parents' views of outcome have been reported.[9 25] As satisfaction is likely to be increased if treatment goals with parents or children, or both, are agreed, a goal attainment rating scale is being tried locally as a first step in this direction, and we are considering making it more "computer game-like" to interest the children.

Acceptability—The local child population is very mixed culturally, with the largest minority ethnic group being Afro–Caribbean.

We have aimed, in the past few years, to make the service more acceptable to ethnic minority families and have undertaken appropriate staff education, appointed more ethnic minority staff members, and offered training specifically to ethnic minority students. Finding appropriate toys is not easy, but is visibly appreciated. There is no longer a marked difference in uptake between the hospital and community provision, whereas previously only the community clinics saw ethnic minority children in numbers proportional to their presence in the population.

Box 1—Issues in consumer research in child psychiatry

Preparatory information for first attendance

Improving attendance rate

Waiting time for assessment

Patient satisfaction with the process and the outcome of treatment

Acceotability of the service, cultural or ethnic sensitivity.

Other health professionals

GPs, hospital and community paediatricians, health visitors, and school nurses can also be customers of child and family psychiatry services. Dissatisfaction can easily arise if there are situations of high risk or distress, or both, and the child psychiatry service seems slow or remote. This can occur not merely through the limitation of resources, but because "child guidance" had until recently little relation with the primary health care system. Improving communication must therefore be a priority, as GPs themselves are making clear.[26]

Information—Referrers' knowledge and expectations of the services of one of the local child guidance units were found to be more accurate than the parents', but still somewhat vague.[17] Leaflets describing clinic services were in popular demand previously, and need updating. There is an active department of general practice, through which other information is disseminated, and occasional "Meet the GP" sessions are arranged.

Letters—Even though many referrals to children's mental health services are not from GPs, there is usually a policy that the GP should be kept informed. Audit of our own practice in this respect showed a frequent deficiency but is now improving.

Liaison—Over the past few years we have increased outreach to GPs[27] and liaison with hospital and community paediatric services including health visitors. The impact of these efforts is difficult to quantify, but they are all subject to review and are dropped if not successful or if other provision becomes available, such as the appointment of a specialist counsellor. Requests for further involvement or for training are encouraging.

Satisfaction—Locally, surveys of GP satisfaction have so far been carried out at hospital and general psychiatric service level only, but elsewhere surveys of the satisfaction of GPs and health visitors with their local child and family psychiatric service have been reported with informative results.[28][29] Such surveys are now being requested by commissioning authorities, and they offer an opportunity to identify deficiencies that may support requests for more resources.

Education and social services

Locally, as with many "child guidance" services, referral has been open to education and social services; clinics were planned, staffed, and administered with the local authorities. Satisfactory relationships with the local authority agencies are therefore crucial to the maintenance of the service, but may not be enough with local government budget pressures and competing statutory priorities.[2]

Social services—Our service offers regular liaison to area offices, arranges meetings at senior level to discuss priorities, offers training courses, and attends committees such as the Area Child Protection Committees and Joint Care Planning Groups. Nevertheless, hospital social work has been subject to freezes and cuts, and unrealistic expectations easily arise with respect to the child psychiatry service's appropriate role in and capacity for child abuse work. (Involvement in child abuse can be a major part of a child mental health service's work, but is exceptionally consuming of resources.[30][31]) "Public relations" work is therefore constantly necessary.

Education—Since the abolition of the Inner London Education Authority the funding for the non-health professionals in the two local child guidance units has been under repeated threat. However, while resources are being put in by education authorites, it is important to work out priorities with them—an example is working to prevent expulsion from school, rather than spending a lot of time on special educational assessments after the event.[32]

Box 2—Methodologies to improve child psychiatry services

Marginal cost benefit analysis

Audit
- team level
- inter-team level
- planning group level

Outcome measures: administrative outcomes
- therapeutic outcome measures
- performance indicators
- health outcomes

Consumer research and quality
- with the child & family
- with other professionals.

The purchasing environment

COMPETITION OR COLLABORATION?

Improving efficiency is a clear aim of the NHS reforms, but the emphasis is more on costing throughput than clinical outcome, and the intended method is that of the market, which can produce distortions.[33][34]

Although many small child psychiatry services are potentially monopoly providers, in a large city such as London purchasers might theoretically invite competitive tenders. There is no obvious "spare" capacity currently, so this would be wasteful of resources as cost differences between services are likely to be partly due to inaccurate allocation of costs, and differences of "case-mix". Encouraging collaboration between adjoining services would be a better strategy for ensuring the availability of a comprehensive but mainly community based service, with some possibility of consumer choice. Standardisation of information collection and quality ratings would be helpful, and some specialisation at different centres might lead to greater efficiency at the margins.

DEMAND AND NEED

Basic epidemiological information is already available in child psychiatry, including knowledge of the social concomitants of childhood disturbance that are more readily measurable.[35-37] "Need" in child psychiatry is usually estimated to be much in excess of potential sources of help, but "needs" are relative and are meaningless without a notion of possibilities of amelioration.[7 38] "Demand" can be very much altered by, for instance, publicising a service, and waiting lists can expand or contract according to the way they are managed. Purchasers should therefore be aware of the relativity of both demand and need.

OBJECTIVES, VALUES, AND PRIORITIES

The purchasers' responsibility is to procure health services offering the best possible value for money for their population. Accepting that resources are always limited, in child psychiatry some "quality values" may have to be traded off against each other: easy accessibility versus carrying out an initial consultant assessment, for instance, or comprehensiveness of case notes against information returns. Choices will have to be made over the use of time—for example, should a court request for assessment take priority over GP referred cases? Should there be more psychological support for terminally ill children and their families, or should there be a specialist team for autistic children? There must be discussion between purchasers and providers about objectives and values, which can lead to the establishment of agreed principles to determine priorities. Priorities should be considered in conjunction with those of the local paediatric and psychiatric services and of GPs. The local authority should also be consulted, to maintain and develop collaborative service arrangements.

Conclusion

In conclusion, the reorganisation of the NHS has produced many challenges, but within it there are also opportunities for rethinking how to make the best use of child psychiatry services to reduce the burden of mental health problems for children now, and for their future adult lives.

1 Department of Health and Social Security. *Fit for the future: report of the Committee on Child Health Services.* Chairman: Professor SDM Court. London: HMSO, 1976. (Court report.)
2 Trowell J. What is happening to mental health services for children and young

people. *Association for Child Psychology and Psychiatry Newsletter* 1991;**14**(5):12–5.

3 Department of Health. *Children Act 1989*. London: HMSO, 1989.

4 Department of Education and Science. *The Education Act 1981*. London: HMSO, 1981.

5 Department of Education and Science. *The Education Reform Act 1988*. London: HMSO, 1988.

6 Department of Health. *Working for patients*. London: HMSO, 1989.

7 Mooney GH, Russell EM, Weir RD. *Choices for health care*. 2nd Ed. London: Macmillan Education, 1986.

8 Royal College of Psychiatrists. Preliminary report on medical audit. *Psychiatric Bulletin* 1989;**13**:577–80.

9 Pound A, Cottrell D. Audit and evaluation in child mental health services. In: Berger M, ed. *Clinic services: monitoring, evaluation and microcomputers*. Association for Child Psychology and Psychiatry. Occasional Papers No 1. London: ACPP 1989:10–4.

10 Rutter M. Psychological therapies: issues and prospects. *Psychol Med* 1982;**12**:723–40.

11 Weisz JR, Weiss B, Alicke MD, Klotz ML. Effectiveness of psychotherapy with children and adolescents: a meta-analysis for clinicians. *J Consult Clin Psychol* 1987;**55**:542–9.

12 Richards H. What do they do at the child guidance? *Association for Child Psychology and Psychiatry Newsletter* 1990;**12**(3):13–7.

13 Cottrell D, Hill P, Walk D, Dearnsly J, Ierothou A. Factors influencing non-attendance at child psychiatry out-patient appointments. *Br J Psychiatry* 1988;**152**:201–4.

14 Walker SR, Rosser RM, eds. *Quality of life: assessment and application*. The Hague: MTP Press, 1988.

15 Nicol AR. Performance indicators in child and adolescent psychiatry. *Psychiatric Bulletin* 1989;**13**:94–7.

16 Jenkins R. Towards a system of outcome indicators for mental health care. *Br J Psychiatry* 1990;**157**:500–14.

17 Subostky F, Berelowitz G. Consumer views at a community child guidance unit. *Association for Child Psychology and Psychiatry Newsletter* 1990;**12**(3):8–12.

18 Burck C. A study of families' expectations and experience of a child guidance unit. *British Journal of Social Work* 1978;**8**:145–58.

19 Garralda ME, Bailey D. Referral to child psychiatry: parent and doctor motives and expectations. *J Child Psychol Psychiatry* 1989;**30**:449–58.

20 Plunkett JW. Parents' treatment expecations and attrition from a child psychiatric service. *J Clin Psychol* 1984;**40**:372–7.

21 Brockless J. The effects of telephone contact prompting on a subsequent attendance at a hospital department of child and adolescent psychiatry. *Association for Child Psychology and Psychiatry Newsletter* 1990;**12**(4):5–8.

22 Mathai J, Markantonakis A. Improving initial attendance to a child and family psychiatric clinic. *Psychiatric Bulletin* 1990;**14**:151–2.

23 Coyle TJ, Paramit KJ, Maisami M. Prospective study of intake procedures in a child psychiatry clinic. *J Clin Psychiatry* 1986;**47**:111–3.

24 Jaffa T, Griffin S. Does a shorter wait for a first appointment improve the attendance rate in child psychiatry? *Association for Child Psychology and Psychiatry Newsletter* 1990;**12**(2):9–12.

25 Thomas H, Hardwick P. An audit of a small child psychiatry clinic. *Association for Child Psychology and Psychiatry Newsletter* 1989;**11**(1):10–4.

26 McGlade KJ, Bradley T, Murphy GJJ, Lundy GPP. Referrals to hospital general practitioners: a study of compliance and communication. *BMJ* 1988;**297**:1246–8.

27 Subotsky F, Brown RM. Working alongside the general practitioner: a child psychiatric clinic in the general practice setting. *Child Care, Health Dev* 1990;**16**:189–96.
28 Markantonakis A, Mathai J. An evaluation of general practitioners' knowledge and satisfaction of a local child and family psychiatric service. *Psychiatric Bulletin* 1990;**14**:328–9.
29 Markantonakis A, Mathai J. An evaluation of health visitors' and social workers' level of knowledge and satisfaction of a local child and family psychiatric service. *Psychiatric Bulletin* 1991;**15**:140–1.
30 Oliver JE. Child protection by child and family guidance workers. *Psychiatric Bulletin* 1991;**15**:197–9.
31 Wressell SE, Kaplan CA, Kolvin I. Performance indicators and child sexual abuse. *Psychiatric Bulletin* 1989;**13**:599–601.
32 Subotsky F. Assessment for special education in a child guidance unit. *Psychiatric Bulletin* 1990;**14**:16–18.
33 Light DW. Effectiveness and efficiency under competition: the Cochrane test. *BMJ* 1991;**303**:1253–4.
34 Quam L. Improving clinical effectiveness in the NHS: an alternative to the white paper. *BMJ* 1989;**299**:488–50.
35 Graham P. Epidemiological studies. In: Quay JC, Werry JS, eds. *Psychopathological disorders of childhood*. 2nd Ed. New York: Wiley, 1979:185–209.
36 Rutter M, Cox A, Rupling C, Berger M, Yule W. Attainment and adjustment in two geographical areas. *Br J Psychiatry* 1975;**126**:493–509.
37 Rutter M, Tizard J, Whitmore K, eds. *Education, health and behaviour*. London: Longman, 1970.
38 Stevens A, Gabbay J. Needs assessment needs assessment... *Health Trends* 1991;**23**(1):20–3.

14. Preventive aspects of child psychiatry

Antony D Cox

The government paper *The Health of the Nation* emphasises disease prevention and health promotion.[1] In the area of mental health it has an objective to reduce ill health and death caused by mental illness, and it states that the mental health of children and adolescents is "a particularly important area as many are vulnerable to physical, intellectual, emotional, social or behavioural developmental disorders which, if not treated, may have serious implications for adult life". There is now plentiful evidence to support this.[2 3] Those who work with children see the prevention and treatment of emotional and behavioural disorders in children as valuable in their own right and not just to prevent adult mental illness. This chapter considers several conceptual issues, indicates contexts in which preventive action may be taken, and cites a number of examples.

Terminology and the goals of prevention

Caplan's categorisation of preventive principles in psychiatry has become popular, but it is somewhat confusing in that it covers what is commonly seen as treatment and rehabilitation as well as prevention.[4] In this categorisation primary prevention aims to reduce the incidence of mental disorders of all types in a community, whereas secondary prevention aims to reduce the duration of an appreciable number of those disorders that do occur. Tertiary prevention is focused on the diminution of impairment resulting from disorders.

Rae Grant helpfully proposes that primary prevention can be seen as covering health promotion and disease prevention,[5] secondary prevention encompasses early identification and treatment, and tertiary prevention is equivalent to rehabilitation. To call all these prevention is to emphasise a "future orientation" and has the advantage that it indicates the indistinct division between primary prevention and treatment.[6]

Newton argues that it is better to draw the line between primary and secondary prevention at a higher level of impairment, that is, at the level of "caseness"—a level of symptomatology approximating to "that of most patients seen by psychiatrists in outpatient settings".[7] Newton argues further that, as preventive work is targeted towards those most vulnerable to disorder, they will probably have some symptoms already. As she emphasises a disease model, she favours a high risk strategy targeted to those most vulnerable to serious mental illness. Preventive intervention "should increase the individual's capacity to control their own life circumstances" and "should make maximum use of existing natural, community and voluntary support networks". Newton's terminology works somewhat better than Caplan's does for child mental health[8 9] and will be adopted in this chapter, which aims to cover a range of activities in primary health care that could certainly be classified as early secondary prevention in Caplan's scheme.

Services and prevention

In developed countries most children with emotional and behavioural disorders (80–90%) do not reach specialist mental health services.[8 10] By no means all of these could be considered as being below "case" level. If specialist services are to be involved then their activities are necessarily indirect, supporting primary health care workers, teachers, and paediatricians. These activities have been covered in some degree by the earlier chapters on consultation and paediatric liaison,[11 12] which are necessarily concerned with both prevention and the treatment of children with substantive emotional and behavioural disorders.

In the case of an individual child it can be academic whether one is concerned with prevention or treatment. What is needed is appropriate working arrangements between primary health care, paediatrics, schools, and the specialist child and adolescent mental health services. However, where resources are scarce more time should be spent on primary prevention and early secondary prevention using organised programmes, as limited resources will be rapidly blocked by severe and intractable cases. This is an appropriate use of resources but is unpopular with many referrers who want difficult problems off their hands.

A conceptual framework

Primary prevention has been considered in a variety of ways and Offord[6] draws attention to the typology emanating from Bloom[13] and Heller et al.[14] This subdivides prevention into community wide, milestone or life transition, and high risk. The focus of prevention may be a combined one, so a programme for all primagravid mothers in a particular community includes both community wide, milestone, and high risk components. Risks can be a facet of an individual or of their environment in the form of chronic stressors or specific experiences, namely life events.[15] Such specific experiences range from personal traumas, as in sexual abuse, to natural disasters.[16]

In the case of children, parents are often the mediators of stressors and indeed may be the stressors themselves. A public health categorisation[6] draws attention to these distinctions. The host or child is the individual at risk while the parent is the agent or environmental medium through which the noxious influence is transmitted—all this occurring in a particular environment, that is ecology or circumstances. Child mental health services are concerned with dysfunctions in relationships as well as symptomatology in individual children. However, terminological confusion is reduced if attempts to improve relationships in the absence of child symptomatology are designated prevention. The child can also be considered as being involved in interlocking systems at different levels: micro-, meso-, exo-, and macro-.[17] The microsystem corresponds to the child's immediate family and the macrosystem to influences at national and international level.

These conceptualisations highlight the manner in which prevention can be focused at different points. Child psychological and psychiatric disorders, however, are not only multifactorial but are generated and sustained by various processes. One model is that the child has particular vulnerabilities and liabilities, as well as assets and resources, and is subject to chronic difficulties in the psychosocial environment such that particular experiences may bring about disorder.[18] The factors can feed into this general model in various ways. For example there can be causal chains or transactional or circular processes.[19–22]

A causal chain would exist when a child with a developmental

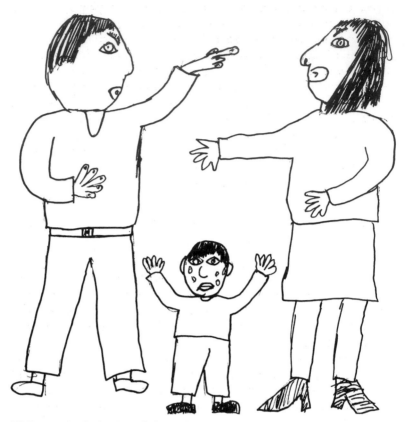

"My parents don't get on." Sometimes children's disturbance is closely linked to family problems

disorder then experiences educational failure, becomes disillusioned with school, plays truant, and becomes delinquent. A transactional process would be when parental unresponsiveness consequent on depression leads a child to be more insistently demanding, which provokes indecisive and hostile parental behaviour. This in turn generates non-compliant child behaviour, which leads to a circular coercive process.[20 23]

Knowledge about common causal chains and transactional and circular processes provides guidance for preventive action. The action can be conceived as primarily focused on reducing personal vulnerability, increasing competence, reducing stressors or their impact, or diminishing the adverse effects of particular experiences. It may also aim to change circular processes by altering communications, roles, perceptions, attitudes, or beliefs.

The part played by specialist child and adolescent mental health professionals can range from direct participation with particular children and families to the promotion of preventive programmes focused on high risk populations, or the role of advocate applying political pressure at a local or national level.[5] Some of those writing about prevention define primary prevention only in terms of programmes as opposed to individually focused approaches.[6] Despite the somewhat blurred distinction between prevention and treatment, there are evidently many opportunities for preventive activity in day to day clinical work.

Problems with primary prevention

The problems that arise are practical, economic, and ethical. Practically, if a child is asymptomatic then the family or others in contact with the child such as the school may be reluctant to engage in a preventive programme. A school may require persuasion to adopt an antibullying campaign. Secondly, intensive programmes may bring about short term change: sustaining change may be more difficult.

If a non-discriminating preventive approach is used, as in some anti-AIDS campaigns, there is a danger that those most in need will not be engaged sufficiently and it will not be possible to modulate the approach according to the needs of different groups.[24] Even if a high risk approach is used there is considerable danger that it will help those who do not require help and fail to reach those in greater need.[24-27] For example the Rochester Primary Mental Health Project aimed to reduce the need for psychiatric treatment among primary grade children identified as having "incipient problems" on the basis of classroom observations, psychological tests, and interviews with the mothers.[28] Not only did the intervention fail to reduce the rate of referral for psychiatric treatment in the index group but the referral rate was less than 20% in the control high risk group. This means that more than 80% of those in the index group had an intervention that they did not need.

Ethical considerations arise because there may be unintended or adverse affects of the intervention,[29] for example through labelling or involvement in inappropriate intervention processes.[30] Is it possible to justify the routine treatment of all children who have

---

Box 1—Reasons for preventive intervention

Child vulnerability
- Genetic counselling for: autism, multiple tics, or bipolar affective illness
- Children with chronic or recurrent physical disability

Chronic difficulties: the child and the family
- Child: low intelligence or emergent psychiatric symptomatology
- Family: social disadvantage or low socioeconomic status, single parents, young mothers
- Vulnerable mother: depression or anxiety, marital difficulties

Life events and experiences
- Naturally occurring life transitions
- Bereavements
- Divorce of parents
- Admission to hospital
- Child sexual abuse
- Teenage pregnancy.

---

been sexually abused, whether or not they are symptomatic? There are somewhat varying reports of the adverse long term consequences of child sexual abuse, and these may relate in part to issues of definition and the need to identify concomitant risk factors.[31][32] This highlights the importance of correct identification of the high risk group and the features responsible for the increased risk.

Focus for preventive intervention

CHILD VULNERABILITY

Genetic counselling

A recent review concludes that childhood autism "is probably quite strongly genetically determined"; that some varieties of multiple chronic tics may be due to a single gene locus, and that major affective disorders with origin in childhood, particularly those of bipolar type, may have a significant genetic component.[33] There are of course a wide variety of genetically determined physical disorders encountered in current paediatric practice that may carry an increased risk for child mental health problems, but genetic counselling in these cases is usually more concerned with the prediction of physical rather than psychiatric disability. Of the disorders encountered in child psychiatric practice it is probably only pervasive developmental disorders, tics, and bipolar affective disorders that require discussion of genetic issues with parents. In autism and related disorders parents may limit their offspring because of the very high heritability that can be presumed in families with other affected individuals.[34]

Children with chronic or recurrent physical disabilities

Children with chronic disease are more likely than healthy children to develop emotional and behavioural disorders.[35] This is particularly true for disorders involving the central nervous system or physical disability. Rates are also higher where there is mental retardation. The impact on family members, both parents and siblings, is increasingly well understood. Preventive work both with regard to the child and to the family, is a component of good paediatric practice.[36]

The manner in which child psychiatrists and psychologists may link up with paediatricians for a wide range of children's physical disorders is described by Leslie (see also the liaison chapter in this book).[11] There is also evidence that a comprehensive counselling approach with children, parents, or families may produce mental health benefits, particularly in individuals where there are additional risk factors.[37]

Davis and Rushton trained parent advisors in basic counselling skills to work with families of children with moderate to severe intellectual or multiple disabilities.[38] Work was initially on a weekly basis but with gradually decreasing frequency over a 15 month period. The aim was to support all members of the family and encourage them to develop a problem solving approach using the family's own resources. There were appreciable improvements in many aspects of family relationships, not just with the index child. For example mothers developed more social contacts and felt more positive about the child, themselves, and their husbands. Compared with the randomly allocated control group, index children made appreciably greater developmental and behavioural progress. This is an approach that has potentially wide applicability in a range of disorders including, for example, asthma and diabetes.

CHRONIC DIFFICULTIES: THE CHILD AND THE FAMILY

For the young child the family constitutes the child's main or sole environment, mediating or buffering wider environmental influences. At a later stage the school and the immediate community have more direct effect. There has been a wide range of preventive programmes in the USA and some in the UK that aim to promote the development of high risk children, either by direct approaches to the child or through the family, or both. High risk for the child has usually been defined in terms of the environment, although in some studies they have been selected because of low intelligence quotient (IQ) or emergent psychological or psychiatric symptomatology. In this latter case the programmes can be considered prevention in Newton's terms and early secondary prevention in Caplan's. The aim of the programmes has varied from promotion of the child's intellectual growth and educational attainment to concern with their emotional development, more particularly the prevention of child abuse and neglect. Variation between programmes and the inclusion of diverse elements in them makes comparisons difficult. For example there is variation in (a) whether the focus is on the child, the parents, or both; (b) whether the intervention has its onset during pregnancy or during primary or secondary school; (c) how long it is sustained; (d) the staff involved who may be specialist, primary health care professionals or volunteers; and (e) the method that may vary not only as to whether the programmes are directed to individuals or groups but also whether the orientation is educational, behavioural, or psychodynamic. There have been several valuable reviews.[5 7 24 39 40]

Who should the programme be directed to?

Seitz drew attention to the greater benefits from programmes for impoverished children that have included family support with or without direct action with the child.[39] Commenting on the report by the Consortium for Longitudinal Studies on 11 Head Start social and cognitive stimulation programmes in the USA for 3–5 year old children from low income families, she pointed out that parents were engaged in virtually all the 11 studies,[41] there being active involvement in more than half the projects. Other projects she reviewed that focused on just the child produced short term IQ gains that tended to wash out and very rarely long term educational or psychosocial benefits. Sometimes there were improvements compared with controls,[42] but there was still a very high rate of educational failure. This was disappointing considering the normal IQs that the children had obtained before entering school. Seitz argues that one of the later preschool programmes, the Perry preschool project,[43] obtained good results because there was a very extensive home visiting programme: 1–1·5 hours a week for 40 weeks a year for two years. The target group consisted of low income and low IQ black children aged 3 and 4.

Of the projects with a more explicit family support model, the Rochester nurse home visitation programme has been among the most successful.[44-46] Women recruited to the project were pregnant with their first child and had one or more of three characteristics: low socio–economic status, age less than 19, or single parent status. Even in this successful project only 80% of the women invited to participate became involved, which emphasises that no project has been successful with all families. Indeed McGuire and Earls have commented on the failure of early preventive intervention programmes to engage all families to point out that it is commonly the families most in need even among disadvantaged groups that are least cooperative.[24] In contrast to Seitz, they advocate a direct approach to the child in these instances. However, they acknowledge the success of the Rochester nurse home visitation project.

In the Rochester programme the most intensively visited group had nine prenatal home visits of 1·25 hours and further visiting for two years postnatally: weekly for the first month after delivery, and then with diminishing frequency to visits at six week intervals. There were lower rates of child abuse, and observational data showed less punishment and restriction of, and greater availability of play materials for, children in the index group. In the highest risk families the children who were visited made the greatest gain in intellectual functioning and the mothers had fewer subsequent pregnancies, returning to school more frequently. Those beyond school age were more likely to get jobs and were less dependent on welfare.

Sylva has turned the focus towards interventions for children outside the home. In a review she concluded that "(a) educationally orientated preschool programmes can prevent cognitive and behavioural problems later in life; (b) the children most at risk of behavioural and intellectual problems attend day care provision; and (c) there is an urgent need to improve educational provision in day nurseries if the 'life chances' of so many disadvantaged children are to be improved".[47]

It is likely that no one approach will engage all families. The experience of the child outside the home should not be neglected—indeed should be used as there is evidence that it can have a protective effect.[48-50] However neither should the family be ignored—sustaining change is a major issue in prevention. A failure to have any impact on the family may have crucial consequences in this regard.[39]

When should the intervention occur?

Intervention in pregnancy and preschool—One project reported by Larson systematically compared the efficacy of home visiting during pregnancy, as opposed to postnatally, in working class Canadian women with healthy babies and no history of admission to psychiatric hospital.[51] The observed quality of maternal interaction with the child was best among those who had had prenatal visits as opposed to those who had only postnatal visits or no visiting prenatally or postpartum. As the improvements in the prenatally visited group were similar to those found in the Rochester nurses home visiting project, it may be that the timing of intervention is crucial as Seitz suggests;[39] Larson's postpartum visited group did not get visits until six weeks after discharge from hospital, whereas the Rochester mothers were visited in the week after delivery.

In the UK Elliot *et al* identified pregnant women as vulnerable to postnatal depression on the basis of a less than satisfactory marital relationship, previous psychological problems, or a high score on a measure of anxiety.[52] Support groups during pregnancy were effective in reducing the rates of postnatal depression in involved mothers. They were less successful in engaging second time mothers who were often more concerned with problems surrounding their first child.

Reviewing the evidence from pregnancy and preschool programmes McGuire and Earls conclude that, although earlier prevention may be more effective, there is a need to sustain any improvements that may have been brought about.[24]

Primary school intervention—The most considerable initiative that tested prevention (in Caplan's terms early secondary prevention) in the UK was the Newcastle study (see chapter 6).[53] Groups of children aged 7–8 years and 11–12 years were selected on the basis that they were above cut off points on behavioural screening measures. For each age group three different interventions were compared using index and control groups: (a) parent counselling combined with teacher consultation by a social worker was used in both age groups, as was (b) group therapy, which was also conducted by social workers but with small groups of children within the school; and (c) teacher aids conducted a compensatory enrichment programme of nurture work in primary schools and in secondary schools teachers used behaviour modification supported by psychologists. Children receiving behaviour modification and group therapy showed appreciably greater benefits than controls on a range of outcome measures and to a lesser extent this was true of the nurture work, but parent counselling combined with teacher consultation did not show benefits. Relative improvements in behaviour at home and school in the group therapy and behavioural treatment children increased with the passage of time but academic improvements were not sustained. Repetition of this work with other high risk primary school children has pointed to the importance of parental resilience as a factor in outcome,[54] especially in protecting against hyperactivity and conduct problems. Whether parental resilience is something that can be promoted by prevention is not known.

Another preventive approach used in primary schools has been daily lessons using "game" activity to develop children's interpersonal cognitive problem solving.[55-57] This approach appears to have been successful with pre-schoolers but the results among primary school children have been less firmly positive.[6] Other child centred school age programmes, including affective education and social skills and assertiveness approaches, are referred to by Rae Grant.[5] Affective education programmes aim to enhance children's social and emotional development by increasing awareness of how feelings influence interpersonal and intrapersonal functioning. Rae Grant comments that results are somewhat mixed and that the programmes have tended to have a narrow focus and brief duration.

Who should do the interventions?

In the UK various preventive projects have been undertaken with children aged under 5, many using health visitors,[9] some using volunteers,[58] and there have been studies of the effects of day care provision.[59] There have been no direct comparisons of the effectiveness of different types of professionals compared with volunteers, although one study has compared family therapy, community support in the form of parallel groups for mothers and toddlers, and behavioural management in the home implemented by specialist health visitors.[60 61] The design does not use a comparison between different types of professionals using the same treatment approach.

Health visitors—Recognition of the high prevalence of emotional and behavioural problems in young children[62] and the unique position of health visitors for contact with families with young children[9] has led to many attempts to train or support health visitors in work with young families; to alleviate maternal depression, to assist mothers in managing children's behaviour problems, and for prevention of child abuse. Approaches have included (a) a year's seminar course for health visitors,[63] (b) a district wide consultation service for health visitors,[64] and (c) support groups providing discussion about mutual families, supervision of the health visitors own work, discussion of formal topics, and discussion of possible referrals.[65 66] The first two of these examples were spearheaded by psychologists and the third by a child psychiatrist.

Other models have used specialist health visitors, and Stevenson identifies three types.[67] The first is based in a specialist mental health service and is an outreach health visitor, functioning like a community child psychiatric nurse. The second is a specialist nurse practitioner with particular skills in the topic of mental health and the management of children's behavioural problems who acts as a teaching consultancy resource for other community health visitors. The third model is intermediate. It recognises that not all health visitors wish to do more intensive psychological work with young families so that a group of specialist health visitors are formed—one within each health visitor unit in a district service—who take referrals from health visitor colleagues and general practitioners.

Despite the evident attractiveness of approaches using health visitors, systematic evaluations using control groups have all been equivocal in terms of benefits to maternal mental health,[60 68 69] mothers' reported ability to manage emotional and behavioural problems, and the level of behavioural problems in the children themselves. Stevenson *et al* attempted to form groups of postnatal mothers in general practice but the group with a sustained take up was a very low proportion of the whole—15%.[69] The aim had been to prevent child abuse by improving mothers' mental state and relationships with their children. This report exemplifies the problem of ensuring engagement with the most needy families where prevention is concerned.

The same investigators went on to attempt early secondary prevention by training health visitors in behavioural techniques in working with families with 3 to 4 year old children showing behavioural problems.[69] Their study and that by Weir and

Dinnick[68] both failed to show appreciable improvements attributable to health visitor intervention.

The third study, referred to above, compared family therapy, parallel mother and toddler groups, and specialist health visitors. It also produced somewhat equivocal results, although the mothers' groups were the most successful in resolving the preschool children's problems.[70]

Probably the most widespread programme is the child development programme based at Bristol University.[71] In this scheme, health visitors are trained to become more aware of the mental health and social problems in the families they see and to appreciate that the child is best helped by promoting a mother's self esteem and competence in furthering the development of her child. There are also two structured interviews the health visitors use, one designed for women who have recently had their first child and the second for those who are experiencing parenting difficulties with a preschool child. Training lasts up to three years and is given to a subgroup of self selected health visitors.

The scheme has now been taken up by 18 health authorities across the UK. Although very positive results are reported, there has been no systematic evaluation using control groups. One commentator considered that claims for the efficacy of the programme in improving children's development and reducing the rate of child abuse are "undermined" by "difficulties in the design and analysis of evaluation data".[72] For example, although the yearly rate of injuries per 1000 children was well under half the national average, health visitors recruiting the first 1000 families (those involved in the evaluation) had instructions to exclude children on child abuse registers. Newton observed health visitors at work in the programme and thought that there was too much emphasis on cognitive skills.[7] Although health visitors have reported that the training improved their understanding of the difficulties faced by mothers and made them more sensitive to their needs and improved job satisfaction, it also made the work more emotionally exhausting.[73] Tensions can arise within a health visiting service if the necessary reorganisation of caseloads means that the specialist health visitors have fewer families to deal with than their colleagues.[7]

The approach using workshops and regular support for health visitors in the New Forest did not prevent referral to the specialist service. On the contrary referral rate increased, but it was thought that referrals became more appropriate.[65 66] An interesting aspect of this particular approach has been the use of joint first visits with health visitors and joint ongoing work. However, there was still a handful of health visitors who had not visited the clinic in the four year period reported on.

Befriending schemes for mothers—Two volunteer schemes that aim to help families with children aged under 5 who are experiencing difficulties in child rearing or are suffering stress are Home-Start and Newpin. Home-Start,[74] the most widespread befriending scheme in the UK, started in Leicester in 1974. In 1990 there were 138 schemes, not only in the UK but in Germany, Canada, Israel, and Australia. Recognising that many families have difficulty rearing young children, the schemes aim to support parents by trained volunteer befrienders. The relationship between volunteer and befriender is central. Local organisations have a paid home start organiser backed by a support group and links to relevant local agencies. The focus is on families with children under 5 and, although the main work occurs in the befriending relationship, many schemes provide a range of other supportive opportunities such as mothers' groups. Volunteers tend to be older and somewhat better educated than those who they are supporting. An uncontrolled evaluation of the project provided very encouraging results[74] with health visitors and families reporting considerable change in more than 80% of instances. Volunteers themselves were the most conservative but even they reported at least some change in more than 80% of cases.

Newpin was set up with an explicit goal to prevent child abuse and neglect.[75] Starting in south London in 1982 it is much less widespread than Home-Start but there are now several centres within and outside London. Each has a paid organiser and administrator, with additional professional input for some group training sessions. The distinction between befriender or volunteer and the mother befriended is not emphasised, and all mothers have the opportunity for personal development work in groups. Those taking on a befriending role also have weekly teaching of a more didactic type over a six month period. The Newpin centre and the ability to drop into it and use the crèche are very important components of the scheme. Initial uncontrolled evaluation pointed to pronounced improvements in the mothers' mental states and in topics that had been identified as a focus of a change, such as maternal isolation or the relationship with the child.[75]

A more rigorous controlled evaluation confirmed the pronounced benefits to the mothers themselves in that virtually all of those engaged in the scheme reported improvements in their mental wellbeing and ability to take charge of their own lives.[76 77] Analysis taking into account duration of involvement in the scheme indicated that improvements in mental state required somewhere between six and 12 months. The relationship with the child was evaluated blind from videotapes of meal and bath times in the home. This very rigorous assessment indicated that improvements in parent–child relationship were more difficult to establish. These occurred in several instances but there were mothers with extended involvement in the scheme, and who had improvements in their own mental health, who still had unsatisfactory relationships with their children. The scheme has now made appropriate modifications to deal with this issue.

Not all mothers were well engaged, and in the period evaluated some 30% dropped out. This appears to reinforce the point made by McGuire and Earls that some of the most needy individuals may not be reached by preventive approaches.[24] However, in the case of Newpin it was those with an intermediate level of difficulty, either in terms of parental mental state or child problems, that tended to drop out; those with more severe problems stayed in. The stringent evaluation of the parent–child relationship has rarely been attempted in the assessment of prevention projects or treatment services.

There is no doubt that volunteer befriending schemes can fill a widespread need.[58] However, different approaches will be required for different families. An established working relationship always needs to exist between such schemes and professional services to effect mutual referral.

What method should be used?

Didactic compared with relationship based methods—Seitz's discussion of this issue has already been referred to in considering who the programme should target. In her review it is difficult to distinguish the person targeted from the approach used—educational or family support.[39] An American project compared two models of family support and found that a didactic approach was less successful than one that focused on relationship building, treating the mother as the person with the responsibility to promote the development of her child.[7 78]

Home compared with day care—Changes in the pattern of family life have emphasised the need to understand the influence of child day care. The quality of care outside the family is clearly crucial, but when day care is meeting certain needs of the child better than at home, the child can benefit.[59] High risk children, however, are not always well served by day nurseries.[79] Not only can the quality of care be important but also the characteristics of the child.[80] Children from impoverished home circumstances gain in social competence and intellectual ability, but results for children's interaction with peers, relationships with their mothers, and compliance with adults are more mixed. Given that those children attending day nurseries in the UK tend to be a high risk population, preventive action in this area is clearly important.[47] One programme to improve the quality of day care is being evaluated in the UK. The programme includes training nursery staff to run art, music, and movement sessions (G Milavic, personal communication, 1992).

Box 2—Short term effects of prenatal and infancy programmes[5]

Children
Better physical health
Better nutrition provided by parents
Fewer low birthweight babies
Fewer feeding problems
Fewer accidents and emergency room to visits
Reduced incidence of child abuse

Parents
Better social support networks
Greater confidence
Improved parenting skills
Better parent–child interactions
More stable marital relationships
Less abuse of children
Longer time periods between pregnancies
More frequent, appropriate use of other services

Short and long term effects of prenatal or infancy programmes

Rae Grant has usefully summarised the short and long term effects of prenatal or infancy programmes,[5] drawing on the high scope Perry preschool programme and other studies in the Consortium for Longitudinal Studies of projects to promote development in under 5 year olds from low income families already referred to (tables I and II).[43 81 82] These impressive results must be viewed

Box 3—Long term effects of prenatal and infancy programmes[5]

Children
    Less aggressiveness and distractability in school
    Less delinquency
    Better attitudes towards school
    Better social functioning
    Higher rates of prosocial attitudes

Parents
    More registration in school by mothers
    More high school completion by mothers
    Higher rates of family employment

with the qualifications given by Setiz[39] and McGuire and Earls[24] that much depends on the nature and quality of the programme. It needs to be oriented to family support as well as to direct intervention with the child, and also to be sufficiently persistent.[40] Some of the most seriously needy individuals may not be engaged. Rac Grant lists the characteristics of effective early childhood programmes[5]:

(1) A developmentally appropriate curriculum based on child initiated activities.

(2) Groups of fewer than 20 children aged 3–5 years with two adults to each group.

(3) Staff trained in early childhood development.

(4) Supervisory support and in service training for the curriculum.

(5) Sensitivity to the non-educational needs of the child and family.

(6) Developmentally appropriate evaluation procedures.

It will be seen that the resource implications are considerable. A major problem with such intensive programmes is generalising them to all needy families in the community.

Children of psychiatrically ill parents

That there is a high risk of emotional and behavioural disorders among children of psychiatrically ill parents is well established.[83 84] Although goals for prevention have been described,[85] namely to improve the stability of the family system, to foster the ability of the mother to meet the children's needs, and to minimise the pathology to which the children are exposed, there have been no systematic studies of interventions to prevent the occurrence of emotional and behavioural disorders in the children. It is clear, as in the case of children in institutions, that the development of positive experiences[48] and the establishment and maintenance of good relationships with either one of the parents or someone outside family can have a protective effect. Similar mechanisms have been shown in the case of marital discord.[49 50] Clearly the preventive interventions described above such as the prenatal intervention to prevent postnatal depression[52] and befriending schemes such as Newpin that aim to improve parental mental health are relevant, but what is needed is the evaluation of a specific programme to benefit children living with a psychiatrically ill parent.

LIFE EVENTS AND EXPERIENCES

Prevention programmes may prepare children in such a way that they avoid unsatisfactory experiences as in the case of sexual abuse, or assist them in coping with the consequences of trauma once it has happened, as in the case of natural disasters. Children who are already vulnerable by virtue of their own characteristics, early experiences, or family environment are most likely to have adverse consequences to noxious life events, so psychological and psychiatric problems after such events may be as much an index of the child's vulnerability as the impact of the event. The connection is obvious for self harm or separation from parents where it is now well established that it is the antecedents, concomitants, and consequences of separation that are of crucial importance in determining the mental health outcome.[86]

Naturally occurring transitions

An example of a preventive programme that attempts to prevent the adverse consequences of naturally occurring transitions is the school transition environment programme that has attempted to reduce the stressful effects of transition to high school.[87 88] This programme involved reorganisation of the school as well as specific interventions with the children themselves. For example the classrooms for children entering the school were arranged to be close to each other so that the new students did not need to adapt to frequent changes in environment and peers. "Home-rooms" were provided for the new pupils where teachers were available to provide counselling and support, some of this on a regular basis. Follow up benefits are said to have included less school failure, behaviour disorders, substance abuse, and delinquency.

Bereavement

This has been much more fully studied in adults, and grief reactions in young children tend to be milder and shorter than in adolescents.[89] However, in a study by Black and Urbanowitz children over 5 who talked within the family about the dead parent within the month after bereavement had a surviving parent who was less likely to be severely depressed or grieving and the children were more likely to have a good psychological outcome a year later.[90]

Divorce

Children are increasingly likely to experience parental separation or divorce. Prevention programmes with the children in these families have been tried out but have not been adequately evaluated.[5] In one such divorce intervention programme, 9–11 year old children were recruited through parents to engage in some 10 or 11 one hour group meetings in the school.[91 92] Each group contained six to nine boys and girls. In the first study a delayed intervention control group was used and in the second study comparison was made with a demographically matched comparison group of children from intact families attending the same school classes. Appreciable improvements in index groups compared with control groups occurred in teachers' ratings of problem behaviours, parents' rating of their children's adjustment, and the children's own ratings of levels of anxiety, but the outcome measures were taken only two weeks after the intervention ended and there was no later follow up.[6]

Admission to hospital

Many studies have shown that children benefit from preparation for admission to hospital.[93–96] Such interventions have been shown to reduce children's distress during and after the admission, and this may partly be because of a reduction in parental anxiety, if a parent is involved in the preparation procedure.[94] There is a review of the prevention of adverse effects of admission to hospital.[97] Eiser mentions several psychological approaches now being used to assist children with basic medical procedures.[35]

Child sexual abuse

Various educational approaches have been used to teach children how to avoid abuse and obtain assistance from adults,[98] and it has been shown that children can be taught these skills,[99] but it is not clear whether they are able to use them in real life. There is also the problem of whether the greatest impact is on children who are already well protected and at low risk for abuse in their own families.[100]

It has been shown that whole school years can be engaged in such prevention programmes, and one study in Dublin has compared parent and teacher instruction with parent and teacher instruction combined with a programme for the children (M Lawlor, personal communication, 1992). The teacher instruction comprised three sessions using lectures, videos, and discussion to give teachers information about child sexual abuse and how to respond to any indications observed or raised by children. The parents attended a parent–teacher meeting and were given basic information about sexual abuse and the children's safety skills programme that ensued. The difficulty that arises is whether the effort involved produces a commensurate benefit. Clearly it would be valuable to know whether it is instruction of the adults that is of more crucial importance than the instruction of the children, but long term follow up of the Dublin study will be needed to establish this.

The treatment of asymptomatic sexually abused children has already been mentioned. Whether treatment should occur will depend on views about long term outcome.[31 32]

Adoption, fostering, and care

The need to support families after placement of children for long term fostering or adoption is very clear.[101] As yet there is no controlled trial of interventions to assist parents and children and ensure the stability of the placement. Such children, particularly those that are fostered, have higher rates of emotional and behavioural difficulties and lower levels of scholastic attainment.[102 103] Thus there is plenty of scope for prevention, although this may be secondary rather than primary in that many of the children already have evidence of emotional and behavioural problems.

There are particularly high rates of emotional and behavioural disorders among children who have experienced institutional care (P Roy, presentation to Royal College of Psychiatrists, London, March 1983).[104–107] These young people are particularly vulnerable at the point of discharge from care and Newton describes one project, the Bradford aftercare team.[7] The project aims to enable young people to deal better with the practical and emotional problems that they face and reduce the need for future social work support. The service tries to establish contact with the young people before they have actually left care. It employs both individual and group work. Although the service was not taken up by all those approached and there have been no attempts to evaluate it, Newton concludes the service may be effective in preventing psychiatric disorder.

Teenage pregnancy

Another particularly vulnerable group are girls experiencing teenage pregnancy. Not all those young women who become pregnant before the age of 21 are necessarily in a high risk group[108] but there are probably a relatively high proportion who can be considered so. Birch found that 40% of pregnant schoolgirls in an inner London borough were already known to the social services and half of these had been in care.[109] Newton[7] describes the St Michael's Hostels[110] in south London as an example of a preventive service for these young mothers, which provides a structured regime including regular sessions with a key worker and support from a resident social worker.

THE COMMUNITY

Housing

There are higher rates of child psychiatric disorder in urban, particularly inner city, areas.[111][112] One contributing factor appears to be the greater risk for disorder in preschool children associated with flats and high rise buildings.[113] This may be partly due to increased risk from maternal depression in these circumstances,[114][115] but also because people feel in less control of their environment in large cities.[112] However, it is also likely that high levels of environmental threat are present in inner city areas. Direct experience of threat or reports of assaults and burglaries were associated with maternal depression and disorder in preschool children in an inner city area.[23] Coleman has shown the features of housing estate design associated with antisocial behaviour in young males who are the major contributor to environmental threat.[116] Where housing design promotes the unimpeded unsupervised movement of young adolescents, vandalism and other antisocial behaviour is more prevalent.

The school

There has been increasing recognition of the part that schools can play in modulating the risk for emotional and behavioural

problems in children and in influencing their academic performance.[112][117][118] The factors in schools that promote children's behaviour and attainment are now well understood, namely high
expectations for work and behaviour, good models of behaviour
provided by teachers, a respect for children and their achievements
with opportunities for them to be involved in the school as an
organisation, clear disciplinary rules with an emphasis on
encouragement of good behaviour and sparing use of punishment,
pleasant working conditions, good teacher–child relationships, and
a supportive coherent structure for teachers. It has proved much
harder to improve schools as organisations.[119][120] However one area
in which there has been considerable success has been bullying.
Approaches were pioneered by Olweus in Norway[121][122] and are
now being promoted by the voluntary organisation Kidscape in the
UK.[123] Components include adults making it plain that bullying is
not to be tolerated and that children's complaints about bullying
will be listened to. Children are encouraged to speak up if they are
bullied, and are given strategies for coping.

In the USA the Yale Newhaven primary prevention project has
been promoted in primary schools since 1968.[124][125] The programme uses a school planning and management team, has a
parent participation programme and a mental health team, and
pays attention to the specific educational needs of children. The
project is reported to have improved academic achievement and
staff and pupil attendance, and it reduced child behavioural
problems and staff turnover. Parent involvement in school activities increased.

The community outside the family

One project has shown that a recreation programme concerned
with the development of skills outside the school and offered to
poor children can reduce vandalism more than that shown in a
comparison housing estate.[126]

Roles for specialist child mental health professionals

It is clear that there are many roles for the specialist child mental
health professional that are concerned with prevention. At the
individual level they may be working on parent–child relationships
in the absence of symptomatology in the child, improving parental
mental health, or working to promote better family function that
may have beneficial effects for siblings, which can be considered as

being preventive even if there is an index symptomatic child. Consultation and liaison roles have already been referred to and in these circumstances there may be a primary prevention role in working with groups of staff who are directly involved with vulnerable children, such as those experiencing chronic physical illness. The teaching role overlaps with both consultation and liaison in that good teaching involves follow through. Ideally there is active discussion of work with particular families in order to reinforce and sustain the effects of any formal teaching.

Child psychiatrists and psychologists have also been involved in facilitating community projects and programmes of the various types described in this chapter. Research evaluation is crucial if there is to be a satisfactory understanding about how to focus preventive efforts economically. Finally there is the advocate role which can be considered relevant to all working with children. It looks to improve the general climate and circumstances, both economic and social, in which children are raised.

Comment

It will be seen that there is very wide range of activities in which specialist child mental health professionals may be engaged that can be considered preventive, encompassing primary prevention and early secondary prevention as defined by Caplan, or simply prevention as defined by Newton. Generally such professionals become involved in high risk prevention rather than that aimed at communities at large. However, some are engaged in activities at community level either directly in prevention of sexual abuse programmes or by advising those who are directly involved.

It continues to be important to understand the nature of the pathological processes so that preventive efforts are focused appropriately. There is a need for effective screening procedures for risk if efforts are not to be wasted. Evaluation is crucial in order to understand the limitations of a preventive intervention not only in terms of what it can achieve but also in terms of those whom it reaches.

There is little doubt that more attention needs to be focused on the development of the resources available to children and protective factors; not confining efforts to the reduction of liabilities and risks. There are many circumstances, for example where a parent is mentally ill, when little can be done in a direct sense about the risk factor, but there is much that can be done protectively in attempting to give children good and satisfying experiences and relationships with others that promote their self esteem.

1 *The health of the nation: a strategy for health in England.* HMSO, 1992.
2 Robins L, Rutter M. *Straight and devious pathways from childhood to adulthood.* Cambridge: Cambridge University Press, 1990.
3 Zeitlyn H. Current interests in child–adult psychopathological continuities. *J Child Psychol Psychiatry* 1990;**31**:671–9.
4 Caplan G. *Principles of preventive psychiatry.* New York: Basic Books, 1974.
5 Rae Grant NI. Primary prevention. In: Lewis M, ed. *Child and adolescent psychiatry: a comprehensive textbook.* Baltimore: Williams and Wilkins, 1991:918–29.
6 Orford J. *Community psychology: theory and practice.* Chichester: Wiley, 1992:154–78.
7 Newton J. *Preventing mental illness in practice.* London: Tavistock/Routledge, 1992.
8 Offord DR. Prevention of behavioural and emotional disorders in children. *J Child Psychol Psychiatry* 1987;**28**:9–19.
9 Stevenson J. Introduction. In: Stevenson J, ed. *Health visitor based services for pre-school children with behaviourproblems.* London: Association for Child Psychology and Psychiatry, 1990:2–6.
10 Rutter M, Tizard J, Whitmore K. *Education health and behaviour.* London: Longman, 1970.
11 Leslie SA. Paediatric liaison. *Arch Dis Child* 1992;**67**:1046–9.
12 Steinberg D. Consultative work in child and adolescent psychiatry. *Arch Dis Child* 1992;**67**:1302–5.
13 Bloom B. The evaluation of primary prevention programs. In: Roberts L, Greenfield N, Miller M, eds. *Comprehensive mental health: the challenge of evaluation.* Madison: University of Wisconsin Press, 1968:117.
14 Heller K, Price R, Reinharz S, Riger S, Wandersman A, D'Aunno T. *Psychology and community charge: challenges for the future.* Homewood, Illinois: Dorsey, 1984.
15 Masten AS. Resilience in development: implications of the study of successful adaptation for developmental psychopathology. In: Cicchetti D, ed. *The Emergence of a discipline.* Hillsdale, NJ: Lawrence Erlbaum, 1989:261–94.
16 Cox A. Social factors in child psychiatric disorder. In: Bhugra D, Leff J, eds. *Principles of social psychiatry.* Oxford: Blackwell, 1992:202–33.
17 Bronfenbrenner U. *The ecology of human development: experiments by nature and design.* Cambridge, Massachusetts: Harvard University Press, 1979.
18 Brown GW, Harris TO, Bifulco A. Long-term effects of early loss of parent. In: Rutter M, Izard CE, Read PB, eds. *Depression in young people: developmental and clinical perspectives.* New York: Guilford Press, 1986:251–96.
19 Gorell Barnes G. Systems theory and family theory. In: Rutter M, Hersov L, eds. *Child and adolescent psychiatry: modern approaches.* Oxford: Blackwell, 1985:216–29.
20 Patterson GR. *Coercive family process.* Eugene, Oregon: Castalia, 1982.
21 Rutter M. Pathways from childhood to adult life. *J Child Psychol Psychiatry* 1989;**30**:23–51.
22 Sameroff AJ, Fiese BH. Transactional regulation and early intervention. In: Meisels SJ, Shankoff JP, etc. *Handbook of early intervention.* Cambridge: Cambridge University Press, 1991:119–49.
23 Cox A, Pickering C, Pound A, Mills M. The impact of maternal depression in young children. *J Child Psychol Psychiatry* 1987;**28**:917–28.

24 McGuire J, Earls F. Prevention of psychiatric disorders in early childhood. *J Child Psychol Psychiatry* 1991;**32**:129–54.

25 Belsky J. Experimenting with the family in the newborn period. *Child Dev* 1985;**56**:376–91.

26 Belsky J. A tale of two variances: between and within. *Child Dev* 1986;**57**:1301–5.

27 Osofsky JD, Culp AM, Ware LM. Intervention challenges with adolescent mothers and their infants. *Psychiatry* 1988;**51**:236–41.

28 Levine M, Perkins D. *Principles of community psychology: perspectives and applications*. New York: Oxford University Press, 1987.

29 Rutter M. Prevention of children's psychosocial disorders: myth and substance. *Pediatrics* 1982;**70**:883–94.

30 Cadman D, Chambers LW, Walter SD, Ferguson R, Johnston N, McNamee J. Evaluation of public health pre-school child development screening; the process and outcomes of a community programme. *Am J Public Health* 1987;**77**:45–51.

31 Jehu D. Long term correlates of child sexual abuse. In: Ouston J, ed. *The consequences of sexual abuse*. London: Association for Child Psychology and Psychiatry, 1990:21–8.

32 Sheldrick C. Adult sequelae of child sexual abuse. *Br J Psychiatry* 1991;**158**(suppl):55–62.

33 Rutter M, Macdonald H, Le Couteur A, Harrington R, Bolton P, Bailey A. Genetic factors in child psychiatric disorders—II. Empirical findings. *J Child Psychol Psychiatry* 1990;**31**:39–83.

34 Bolton P, Rutter R. Genetic influences in autism. *International Review of Psychiatry* 1990;**32**:85–98.

35 Eiser C. Psychological effects of chronic disease. *J. Child Psychol Psychiatry* 1990;**32**:85–98.

36 Graham P. Psychiatric aspects of pediatric disorders. In: Lewis M, ed. *Child and adolescent psychiatry: a comprehensive textbook*. Baltimore: Williams and Wilkins, 1991:977–94.

37 Davis H, Fallowfield L. Evaluating the effects of counselling and communication. In: Davis H, Fallowfield L., eds. *Counselling and communication in health care*. Chichester: Wiley, 1991:287–318.

38 Davis H, Rushton R. Counselling and supporting parents of children with developmental delay: a research evaluation. *J Ment Defic Res* 1991;**35**:89–112.

39 Seitz V. Intervention programs for impoverished children: a comparison of educational and family support models. *Annals of Child Development* 1990;**7**:73–103.

40 Farran DC. Effects of intervention with disadvantaged and disabled children: a decade review. In: Meisels SJ, Shonkoff JP, eds. *Handbook of early intervention*. Cambridge: Cambridge University Press, 1991:501–39.

41 Lazar I, Darlington R. Lasting effects or early education: a report from the consortium for longitudinal studies. *Monographs of the Society for Research in Child Development* 1982:47. (2–3, Serial No 195.)

42 Horacek HJ, Ramey CT, Campbell FA, Hoffman RP, Fletcher RH. Predicting school failure and assessing early intervention with high-risk children. *J Am Acad Child Adolesc Psychiatry* 1987;**26**:758–63.

43 Berrueta-Clement JR, Schweinhart LJ, Barnett WS, Epstein AS, Weikart DP. *Changed lives: the effects of the Perry preschool programme on youths through age 19*. Ypsilanti, MI: High/Scope Educational Research Foundation, 1984.

44 Olds DL, Henderson CR, Chamberlain R, Tatelbaum K. Preventing child abuse and neglect: a randomised trial of nurse home visitation. *Pediatrics* 1986;**78**:65–78.

45 Olds DL, Henderson CR, Tatelbaum R, Chamberlain R. Improving the

delivery of prenatal care and outcome of pregnancy: a randomized trial of nurse home visitation. *Pediatrics* 1986;77:16–28.

46 Olds DL, Henderson CR, Tatelbaum R, Chamberlain R. Improving the life-course development of socially disadvantaged mothers: a randomized trial of nurse home visition. *Am J Public Health* 1988;78:1436–45.

47 Sylva K. Does early intervention work? *Arch Dis Child* 1989;64:1103–4.

48 Quinton D, Rutter M. Parenting behaviour of mothers raised 'in care'. In: Nicol AR, ed. *Longitudinal studies in child psychology and psychiatry.* Chichester: Wiley, 1985:157–201.

49 Jenkins JM, Smith MA, Graham PJ. Coping with parental quarrels. *J Am Acad Child Adolescent Psychiatry* 1989;28:182–9.

50 Jenkins JM, Smith MA. Factors protecting children living in disharmonious homes: maternal reports. *J Am Acad Child Adolesc Psychiatry* 1990;29:60–9.

51 Larson C. Efficacy of prenatal and postpartum home visits on child health and development. *Pediatrics* 1980;66:191–7.

52 Elliot SA, Sanjack M, Leverton TJ. Parents groups in pregnancy; a preventive intervention of post-natal depression. In: Gottlieb BH, ed. *Marshalling social support.* London: Sage, 1988.

53 Kolvin I, Garside RF, Nichol AR, Macmillan A, Wolstenholme F, Leitch IM. *Help starts here: the maladjusted child in the ordinary school.* London and New York: Tavistock, 1981.

54 Kolvin I, Charles G, Nicholson K, Fleeting M, Fundundis T. Factors in prevention in inner-city deprivation. In: Goldberg D, Tantam D, eds. *The public health impact of mental disorder.* Toronto: Hogrefe and Huber, 1990:112–23.

55 Spivack G, Shure M. *Social adjustment of young children: a cognitive approach to solving real-life problems.* San Francisco: Jossey-Bass, 1979.

56 Shure M, Spivack G. Interpersonal cognitive problem and primary prevention. Programming for pre-school and kindergarten children. *Journal of Clinical Child Psychology* 1979;8:89–94.

57 Shure M, Spivack G. Interpersonal problem-solving in young children: a cognitive approach to prevention. *Am J Community Psychol* 1982;10:341–56.

58 Cox A. Befriending young mothers. *Br J Psychiatry* 1993 (in press).

59 Hennessy E, Melhuish EC. Early day care and development of school-age children: a review. *Journal of Reproductive and Infant Psychology* 1991;9:117–36.

60 Nicol AR, Stretch DD, Davidson I, Fundundis T. Controlled comparison of three interventions for mother and toddler problems: a preliminary communication. *J R Soc Med* 1984;77:488–91.

61 Koziarski M, Hodgson S, Nicol AR. Family therapy in a community mother and toddler project. *Journal of Family Therapy* 1986;8:207–24.

62 Richman N, Stevenson J, Graham P. *Pre-school to school: a behavioural study.* London: Academic Press, 1982.

63 Appleton P, Pritchard P, Pritchard A. *Evaluation of a 12 month in-service course for health visitors in behavioural intervention methods with infants and pre-school children.* Clwyd Health Authority, 1988.

64 Hewitt KE, Crawford WV. Resolving behaviour problems in pre-school children. Evaluation of a workshop for health visitors. *Child Care Health Dev* 1988;14:1–9.

65 Thompson MJJ, Bellenis C. A joint assessment and treatment service for the under fives. *Newsletter of the Association for Child Psychology and Psychiatry* 1992;14:221–7.

66 Bellenis C, Thompson MJJ. A joint assessment and treatment service for the under fives—work with health visitors in a child guidance clinic—part 2 work done and outcome. *Newsletter of the Association for Child Psychology and Psychiatry* 1992;14:262–6.

67 Stevenson J. A summary of his study group's conclusions. In: Stevenson J, ed. *Health visitor based services for pre-school children with behaviour problems.* London: Association for Child Psychology and Psychiatry, 1990:38–40.

68 Weir IK, Dinnick S. Behaviour modification in the treatment of sleep problems in young children; a controlled trial using health visitors as therapists. *Child Care Health Dev* 1988;**14**:355–68.

69 Stevenson J, Bailey V, Simpson J. Feasible intervention in families with parenting difficulties: a primary prevention perspective on child abuse. In: Browne K, ed. *The prediction and prevention of child abuse and neglect.* Chichester: Wiley, 1988:121–38.

70 Nicol AR, Stretch DD, Fundudis R. Pre-school children in troubled families: approaches to intervention and support. Chichester: Wiley, 1993 (in press).

71 Barker W, Anderson R. *The child development programme: an evaluation of process and outcomes.* (Evaluation document 9.) Bristol: University of Bristol, Early Child Development Unit. School of Applied Social Studies, 1988.

72 Stevenson J. The evaluation of collaborative services with health visitors for pre-school children with behaviour problems. In: Stevenson J, ed. *Health visitor based services for pre-school children with behaviour problems.* London: Association for Child Psychology and Psychiatry, 1990:23–31.

73 Child Development Project. *Child development programme.* Bristol: University of Bristol, 1984.

74 Van der Eyken W. *Home-start: a four-year evaluation.* Leicester: Home-Start Consultancy, 1990.

75 Pound A, Mills M. A pilot evaluation of Newpin. *Newsletter of the Association of Child Psychology and Psychiatry* 1985;**70**:13–5.

76 Cox AD, Pound A, Pickering C. Newpin: a befriending scheme and therapeutic network for carers of young children. In: Gibbons J, ed. *The children act 1989 and family support.* London: HMSO, 1992:37–47.

77 Cox AD, Pound A, Mills M, Pickering C, Owen AL. Evaluation of a home visiting and befriending scheme: Newpin. *J R Soc Med* 1991;**84**:217–20.

78 Barnard KE, Hammond M, Mitchell SK, Booth CL, Spietz A, Snyder C, Elsas T. Caring for high risk infants and their families. In: Green M, ed. *The psychological aspects of the family.* Lexington, Massachussets: DC Heath, 1985.

79 McGuire J. Social interactions of young, withdrawn children in day nurseries. *Journal of Reproductive and Infant Psychology* 1991;**9**:169–79.

80 Clarke-Stewart KA. Does day care affect development? *Journal of Reproductive and Infant Psychology* 1991;**7**:67–78.

81 Consortium for Longitudinal Studies. *As the twig is bent.* . . . Hillsdale, NJ: Lawrence Erlbaum, 1983.

82 Woodhead M. When psychology informs public policy: the case of early childhood intervention. *Am Psychol* 1988;**43**:443–54.

83 Cox A. Maternal depression and impact on children's development. *Arch Dis Child* 1988;**63**:90–5.

84 Rutter M. Psychiatric disorders in parents as a risk factor for children. In: Shaffer D, Phillips I, Enzer NB, eds. *Prevention and mental disorders, alcohol and other drug use in children and adolescents.* Rockville, Maryland: Office of Substance Prevention, US Department of Health, 1989:157–89.

85 Goodman SH, Isaacs ID. Primary prevention with children of severely disturbed mothers. *Journal of Preventive Psychiatry* 1984;**2**:387–402.

86 Rutter M. *Maternal deprivation reassessed.* Harmondsworth: Penguin, 1981.

87 Felner RD, Adan AA. The school transitional environmental project: an ecological intervention and evaluation. In: Price RH, Cowen EL, Lorion RP, et al, eds. *14 ounces of prevention.* Washington, DC: American Psychological Association, 1988:111–22.

88 Felner RD, Primavera J, Cauce AM. The impact of school transition: a focus for preventive efforts. *Am J Community Psychol* 1981;9:449–59.
89 Rutter M. The developmental psychopathology of depression: issues and perspectives. In: Rutter M, Izard CE, Read PB, eds. *Depression in young people: clinical and developmental perspectives.* New York: Guilford, 1986:3–30.
90 Black D, Urbanowitz MA. Family intervention with bereaved children. *J Child Psychol Psychiatry* 1987;28:467–76.
91 Pedro-Carroll J, Cowen E. The children of divorce intervention programme: an investigation of the efficacy of a school-based prevention program. *J Consult Clin Psychol* 1985;53:603–11.
92 Pedro-Carroll J, Cowen E, Hightower A, Guare J. Preventive intervention with latency-aged children of divorce: a reflective study. *Am J Community Psychol* 1986;14:277–90.
93 Wolfer JA, Visintainer MA. Pre-hospital psychological preparation for tonsillectomy patients: effects on children's and parents' adjustment. *Pediatrics* 1979;64:646–55.
94 Ferguson BF. Preparing young children for hospitalisation: a comparison of two methods. *Pediatrics* 1979;64:656–64.
95 Cassell S, Paul MU. The role of puppet therapy on the emotional responses of children hospitalised for cardiac catheterisation. *J Pediatrics* 1965;71:233–9.
96 Skipper J, Leonard R. Children, stress and hospitalisation: a field experiment. *J Health Soc Behav* 1968;9:275–87.
97 Byrne CM, Cadman D. Prevention of the adverse effects of hospitalisation in children. *Journal of Preventive Psychiatry* 1987;3:167–90.
98 Gough D. Approaches to child abuse prevention. In: Browne K, Davis C, Stratton P, eds. *Early prediction and prevention of child abuse.* Chichester: Wiley, 1988: 107–20.
99 Fryer GE, Kraiser SK, Miyoshi T. Measuring actual reduction of risk to child abuse: a new approach. *Child Abuse Negl* 1987;11:173–9.
100 Gough DA, Taylor JR, Boddy FA. *Child abuse interventions: a review of the research literature, part B, preventing abuse.* London:Report to DHSS, 1987.
101 Rushton A. Post-placement services for foster and adoptive parents-support, counselling or therapy? *J Child Psychol Psychiatry* 1989;30:197–204.
102 Wolkind S, Rutter M. Children who have been 'in-care'—an epidemiological study. *J Child Psychol Psychiatry* 1973;14:97–105.
103 Rowe J, Cain H, Hindleby M, Keane A. *Long-term foster care: child care policy and practice.* London: Batsford, 1984.
104 Wolkind S. Sex differences in the aetiology of antisocial disorders in children in long-term residential care. *Br J Psychiatry* 1974;125:125–30.
105 Wolkind S, Rutter M. Separation loss and family relationships. In: Rutter M, Hersov L, eds. *Child and adolescent psychiatry: modern approaches.* Oxford: Blackwell, 1985:34–57.
106 Hodges J, Tizard B. IQ and behavioural adjustment of ex-institutional adolescents. *J Child Psychol Psychiatry* 1989;30:53–75.
107 Hodges J, Tizard B. Social and family relationships of ex-institutional adolescents. *J Child Psychol Psychiatry* 1989;30:77–97.
108 Phoenix A. *Young mothers.* Cambridge: Polity, 1991.
109 Birch D. *Schoolgirl pregnancy in Camberwell.* London: University of London. (MD thesis).
110 Pettigrew S. *Building on experience in St Michael's Fellowship.* London: St Michael's Fellowship, 1987.
111 Richman N. Disorders in pre-school children. In: Rutter M, Hersov L, eds. *Child and adolescent psychiatry: modern approaches.* Oxford: Blackwell, 1985:336–50.
112 Wolkind S, Rutter M. Socio–cultural factors. In: Rutter M, Hersov L, eds.

Child and adolescent psychiatry: modern approaches. Oxford: Blackwell, 1985:82–100.

113 Quinton D. Urbanism and mental health. *J Child Psychol Psychiatry* 1988;**29**:11–21.

114 Richman N. Behaviour problems in pre-school children. *Br J Psychiatry* 1977;**131**:523–7.

115 Brown GW, Harris T. *The social origins of depression.* London: Tavistock, 1978.

116 Coleman A. *Utopia on trial: vision and reality in planned housing.* London: Hilary Shipman, 1985.

117 Rutter M, Maughan B, Mortimore P, Ouston J, Smith A. *Fifteen thousand hours—secondary schools and their effects on children.* London: Open Books, 1979.

118 Maughan E. School experiences as risk/protective factors. In: Rutter M, ed. *Studies of psychosocial risk: the power of longitudinal data.* Cambridge: Cambridge University Press, 1988:200–20.

119 Maughan B, Pickles A, Rutter M, Ouston J. Can schools change? I: Outcomes at six London secondary schools. *School Education and School Improvement* 1990;**1**:188–210.

120 Ouston J, Maughan B, Rutter M. Can schools change? II: Practice in six London secondary schools. *School Education and School Improvement* 1991;**2**:3–13.

121 Olweus D. Familial and temperamental determinants of aggressive behaviour in boys: a causal analysis. *Developmental Psychology* 1980;**16**:644–65.

122 Olweus D. Bullying among school boys. In: Barnes R, ed. *Children and violence.* Stockholm: Academic Literature, 1980.

123 Elliott M. A whole-school approach to bullying. In: Elliott M, ed. *Bullying: a practical guide to coping for schools.* Harlow: Longman, 1991:166–75.

124 Comer JP. Improving the quality and continuity of relationships in two inner-city schools. *J Am Acad Child Psychiatry* 1976;**15**:535–45.

125 Comer JP. *School power: implications of an intervention project.* New York: Free Press, 1980.

126 Jones MB, Offord DR. Reduction in antisocial behaviour in poor children by nonschool skill-development. *J Child Psychol Psychiatry* 1989;**30**:737–50.

Index